Fundamentals of Emergency Medical Services System Evaluation and Quality Improvement

Craig A. Stroup
Center for EMS Performance Improvement

Copyright ISBN#
www.cemspi.org

TABLE OF CONTENTS

TABLE OF CONTENTS

EMS Quality Improvement
The Big Picture

Reaching for excellence in any system requires a functional decision making process among the team of workers and users within that system. Inherent to this process is the need to know how the system is functioning and what to do to fix or improve it. The concept of continuous quality improvement (CQI) particularly in the field of prehospital care relies mainly upon the following fundamental components;

1. The availability of reliable and trusted information.
2. The ability to effectively communicate that information in easy to understand ways.
3. A standardized approach to reaching decisions and acting on those decisions.

CQI is best accomplished by improving processes in which people work and not just correcting the shortcomings of the people doing the work. An effective method for getting the job done is to eliminate inefficiencies and ensure that quality is built into the way things are done. This means looking at out-of-date systems and processes – replacing old-fashioned methods with new methods that get the appropriate results. Through continuous quality improvement, the gap will narrow between performance and expectations. It will push the standards upward that will result in better outcomes. Staff should be competent to follow processes and procedures so that things are done correctly. In the clinical area, doing the right things right is analogous to doing appropriate things effectively. Understanding the variability of processes is a key to improving quality. In health care, there are uncontrollable variations related to differences among individuals, organ systems, and diseases. Quality improvement stresses understanding complex processes, measuring performance using reliable statistical methods, and using that information to build quality into our process.

This book is intended to be a supplement to a basic CQI introductory training program with the focus on evaluating and improving emergency medical services (EMS). In our approach, we recognize and distinctly separate our CQI activities into three major components. Specifically, we choose to look at the following as separate but related components of a CQI program;

Component I:	System Evaluation
Component II:	Quality Improvement Initiatives
Component III:	Patient Safety

We have chosen to separate these components because we strongly believe that in order to reach decisions and make quality changes, the process of system evaluation must be done first and done well. Once we have clearly and reliably reached consensus on what we want to measure and how we want to measure it, then and only then should we make decisions about performance and apply the second component of traditional Plan-Do-Check-Act (PDCA) cycle that is inherent to a good classical quality improvement process.

Finally, we separate our comprehensive CQI plan to include a third component; the component we call "EMS Patient Safety". Distinguishing patient safety from the other two components is necessary because it often implies an immediate intervention and the possibility of an action directly affecting a single adverse event, provider or patient.

It could also involve more stringent improvement steps and the possibility of complicated personnel or licensing issues. Since these attributes could conflict with the positive principles and reinforcement of quality improvement theory, it is highly recommended that patient safety be handled separately and clearly apart in both organizational structure and processes from all other system based CQI activities and initiatives.

History and Heroes in Quality

In order to understand what quality is, we must first look at where quality has been and who helped to bring the theories of quality improvement to the forefront in our world and our country. As the great philosopher Santayana once said; "Those who fail to learn from history are condemned to repeat it." No discussion about quality improvement would be complete without first mentioning some of the people who came before us and left us with the keys to being successful. It is very important to have a good base knowledge of where all this "quality" stuff came from and who was instrumental in making it happen. I will just briefly mention some of the pioneers in the basic concepts of quality leading up to the contemporary primary achievements that has helped bring the concepts of quality management in EMS to the front doorstep.

William Deming
Considered by many to be the "father" of quality is William Deming. He was an American engineer, statistician, professor, author, lecturer, and management consultant who first put forward the concepts of quality in industry and the workplace. He is known best by his fourteen points of quality which are hallmark principles integrated into almost all contemporary the following are the fourteen (14) points;

1. Create a constant purpose toward improvement.
2. Adopt the new philosophy.
3. Stop depending on inspections.
4. Use a single supplier for any one item.
5. Improve constantly and forever.
6. Use training on the job.
7. Implement leadership.
8. Build Trust and Drive out Fear.
9. Break down barriers between departments.
10. Get rid of unclear slogans.
11. Eliminate management by objectives.
12. Remove barriers to pride of workmanship.
13. Implement education and self-improvement.
14. Make "transformation" everyone's job.

Joseph Juran
Juran was a Romanian-born American engineer and management consultant. He is principally remembered as an evangelist for quality and quality management, having written several influential books on those subjects. He is most famous for developing the concept of "blame the process not the person"

In 1941, Juran stumbled across the work of Wilfredo Pareto and began to apply the Pareto principle to quality issues (for example, 80% of a problem is caused by 20% of the causes). This is also known as "the vital few and the trivial many". In later years, Juran preferred "the vital few and the useful many" to signal the remaining 80% of the causes should not be totally ignored

Malcolm Baldrige, Jr.
Baldrige was an American politician. He served as the United States Secretary of Commerce from 1981 until his death in 1987 The Malcolm Baldrige National Quality Award is the national quality award that recognizes U.S. organizations in the business, health care, education, and nonprofit sectors for performance excellence.

The Baldrige Criteria for Performance Excellence serve two main purposes; to help organizations assess their improvement efforts, diagnose their overall performance management system, and identify their strengths and opportunities for improvement.

Donald M. Berwick
Berwick was President and CEO of the Institute for Healthcare Improvement (IHI) for nearly 20 years. In July 2010, President Obama appointed Dr. Berwick to the position of Administrator of the Centers for Medicare & Medicaid Services, a position he held until December 2011. Improving the U.S. health care system requires simultaneous pursuit of three aims: improving the experience of care, improving the health of populations, and reducing per capita costs of health care. Preconditions for this include the enrollment of an identified population, a commitment to universality for its members, and the existence of an organization (an "integrator") that accepts responsibility for all three aims for that population.

EMS History
In 1992, the American College of Emergency Physicians (ACEP); published the first national recognized book to address the concepts of applying CQI to EMS called; Continuous Quality Improvement in EMS. The next year in 1993, the National Assn of EMS Physicians, led by Robert Swor who published; Quality Management in Prehospital Care. Both of these publications helped immensely in introduce and translate CQI into the rank and file EMS organizations throughout the nation. In 1997, the National Highway Traffic and Safety Administration (NHTSA): issued their publication; "Emergency Medical Services Agenda for the Future" which included CQI as a separate and distinct part of a functioning EMS system.

National Highway Traffic and Safety Administration (NHTSA)
In 1998, NHTSA published; A Leadership Guide to Quality Improvement for Emergency Medical Services Systems. This document helped set the baseline principles applied to an EMS system in the U.S.

California EMSA Model Guidelines for EMS QI
In 2001, the California Vision Project produced and published one of the first written guidelines that specifically applied to EMS quality improvement programs. To his day it continues to be a great resource for writing and establishing the structure and processes for an EMS CQI program.

Customer Valid Requirements

<u>The Customer</u>
Our customers should be our greatest heroes. EMS service providers whether public or privately must first and foremost keep in mind that excellence in quality means pleasing customers who in turn return the favor by supporting, utilizing and ultimately help the organization to flourish.

Quality is best defined by the customer who includes system stakeholders and subject experts. A common mistake of beginning organizations is to decide behind closed doors what the quality of their services will be without first getting input from their customers. It is important to remember that the customer or in the case of EMS, the patient is the ultimate receiver of products or services. EMS like most industries should clearly identify who their customers are and their expectations. Looking at the customer through the eyes of quality, EMS can analyze the value of their services by recognizing both the obvious and not so obvious recipients of these services. In quality circles, we call this acknowledging the internal and external customers. Below is a short summary of both internal and external customers in typical EMS systems.

EMS Customers	Description	Examples
Internal	Direct recipients or end-users of the services you provide.	Patients, Public
External	Indirect recipients of the services you provide or fellow peers, along the chain of service.	ED Nurses, Physicians, Dispatchers, Clerks, Peers, Regulatory agencies

In the same way, those external customers that you serve should also look at you as a customer. All data collected and measured should be customer (patient) service oriented. Identifying the customer first, followed by defining what their greatest needs are and then realizing what type of information you need to collect and how it should be measured.

Sadly, few organizations take the time to understand how to please their internal and external customers. EMS is particularly vulnerable to this weakness because many of our customers need us and in some ways "have" to call 911 in order to get help. In business this is often called the "spider web" customer because they are "caught" in the web and do not have any other choice but to use our services. While this may work for long periods of time, studies show that all groups of customers and end users trend more toward becoming smarter users as opposed to dumber and dumber users.

Sooner or later even those in public and "essential" service find themselves competing for survival not because they have become ono-essential but because they have ignored their customer base requirements and failed to provide increasingly better quality. When this happens, we the stronger more customer "conditioned" provider slowly takes over because the customer/patient wants what are best and most efficient.

In order to determine the truth about valid customer requirements, we must go to the customer. The truth is we can't know what the customer wants until we ask them. So the first requirement is to have access to the feedback you need to determine their requirements.

The two most common method of obtaining direct input (the truth) from your customers is through the application of regular surveys and meeting face to face with what we have called a consumer review board (CRB). The CRB is made up of volunteer citizens that have been patient/customers The following are the minimum number of issues/questions to help formulate "Valid Customer Requirements" that every organization should ask or survey from their customers (both external and internal) before they formulate a mission statement, performance objectives, and ultimately their CQI plan.

Determining Valid Customer Requirements
They following are key questions to help narrow determine valid customer requirements with an EMS service.

1. What is the primary service we provide?
2. How well are we providing it?
3. What are the most important parts of our service?
4. How well are we providing them?
5. What parts of our service can we improve?
6. How can we improve these parts of service?

Once these questions are answered, they can be narrowed down and reviewed by the organization to determine if they can practically and fiscally implemented. This provides the root-basis for the improvement objectives within the organizations CQI plan. As a provider of services, you are the expert at knowing how to provide for your customers. But your customers are best at knowing what services are needed and why they are needed. There are many more questions to ask specific to your role and the feedback you get from your customers. This process of asking and getting answers back from your customers is the root method for both determining your initial valid customer requirements and modifying or replacing them as time goes on.

If organizations fail to examine and act on their customer needs and opportunities to improve customer based services and processes, they may be left behind by their competition. Customers often have choices and will choose to go elsewhere for their goods and services if they feel dissatisfied or that the services were inferior to others. It is the health care professionals who in the end make the difference by becoming involved in making the health care environment a safer environment where we do the right things as well as doing things right.

EMS Organizational Structure

Program Structure
Below illustrates one of the recommended organizational structures of a typical EMS CQI program (EQIP). Each QIP should have the three distinct branches within the organization, each with separate mission, goals and objectives and each branch driving the whole program forward.

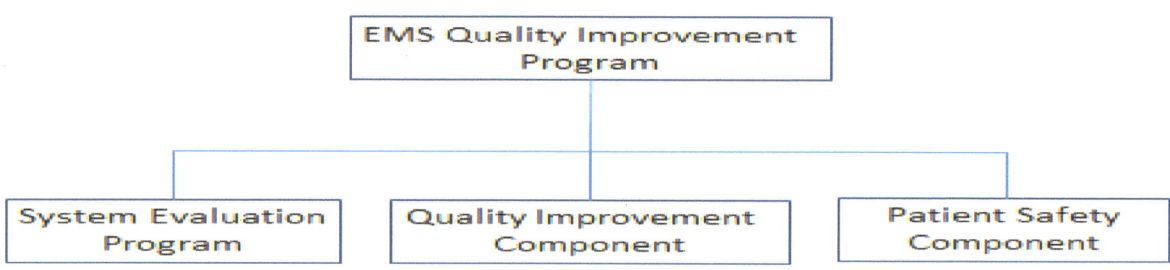

System Structure
A QIP should have a clear understanding of how it integrates and functions within the governmental hierarchy. Below is an organizational chart depicting the integration and hierarchy within the typical EMS system.

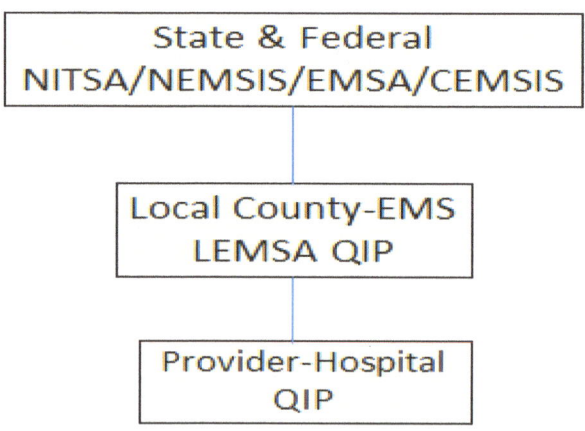

EMS Roles & Responsibilities

CQI programs should have a shared leadership structure and vision made up of a collaborative relationship between our providers, hospitals and EMS agency. All organizations work together through our Quality Leadership Council structure.

The EMS Quality Manager under the direction of the EMS Director and Medical Director provides primary coordination and leadership of all components and committee actions. The following are typical CQI roles and responsibilities within an EMS system. Actual job descriptions for these positions can be found in the appendix of this textbook.

CQI Quality Manager

The Quality Manager is the primary leadership role in any organized quality program. This position is responsible for the overall coordination and activities related to all there components of the system; evaluation, improvement and safety. This position requires a strong formal education and training in the three areas of quality. Experience within the respective CQI program system is very valuable. The manager should have strong analytical, communication and team building skills. Leadership through consensus building also is also a priority skill. This position is often filled by a Physician, Registered Nurse or Paramedic. The Quality Manager may also be the Medical Director if qualified.

CQI Medical Director

This position is usually filled by a physician who has completed a basic course of training in EMS System Evaluation and Quality Improvement (CQI) training as approved by the employing agency.

Data System Manager

This role is primarily to work with the Quality manger and CQI groups to help develop and implement important CQI level measures. This position is a person who has been trained and has demonstrated competency in the overall data system management and who shall be responsible to implement, maintain, troubleshoot, operate, query and produce reports for the data systems which support the contractor's day to day CQI program operations. The Data System Manager shall report to the Quality Manager.

Program Support Staff

Each program should have a sufficient in number and allotted time to fully support day to day operational activities as required providing timely completion of all CQI program activities.

Field Training Officers (FTO)
Each program should have FTOs with a minimum of four (4) years of full time experience in a 911 response system and complete a basic level training course in EMS System Evaluation and Quality Improvement approved by the EMS Agency. The FTO shall be appointed by the provider service and be approved by the Medical Director of the EMS agency.

Local EMS Agency
The EMS agency Medical Director provides the primary decision making role in the county-wide CQI process. In most cases, consensus of all leadership is sought in all decisions related to CQI program activities. Ultimately, if consensus cannot be agreed, final statutory responsibility and ultimately all medical decisions fall to the EMS Medical Director.

Quality Leadership Council (QLC)
The CQI program functions under the control of the EMS agency but through the input and advisory capacity of the QLC. The QLC provides the community leadership and participation to execute all quality evaluations, planning and implementation. The QLC is made up of representatives of all entities directly and indirectly involved in patient care in the prehospital setting. Customer and patient representatives are also included in many of these committees.

Education and Qualifications
Each CQI program should strive to assure that all members have a baseline of knowledge and are familiar with the nomenclature and operations inherent to the CQI culture. Standardized training in EMS system evaluation and improvement should at a minimum be provided and if possible, required for participants

Training
A critical part of developing a robust and productive organization is strong leadership that Communicates and promotes through ongoing training of its leadership and members. Keeping all on the same page and making sure the standardized training is available periodically to update and provide consistency is key to long term effectiveness and accountability in an organized CQI system

Professional Accreditation in EMS Quality
It has only been in recent years that the EMS Industry has begun to recognize the value of standardized training for their quality professionals. While there are standardized training programs in California that have been built specifically for the EMS Industry, there still remains much more to be done. Leadership organizations are now talking about standardized training processes and perhaps even an "accreditation" process to further standardize and professionalize the EMS Quality Manger. In the near future, it may be an industry standard that national quality organizations such as the IHI will begin to specialize EMS quality training and validate this education as an industry standard.

Snakes in the Grass

Some of the progress made in quality and in particular to EMS has been hard fought. Some of the ideas surfacing out of the traditional experiences of quality in U.S. history have been slow to be accepted in the medical disciplines. The following are just some examples of CQI concepts that seem to sometimes have a square shape when it comes time to put them into the circular shaped EMS silo.

Hard vs. Soft Science

While CQI programs strive to provide valuable and real time information, it is NOT held to the same rigors and discipline of traditional scientific research. CQI is often better described as "soft science" that tends to provide a basis or recognition that change may be needed. This is an important distinction. Another major difference is that the CQI information and how it is measured should come from the people or organizations that generate the data and they should trust what was put together. Standardized quality indicators should be the tools that define the data, communicate the information, establish the consensus, stimulate the discussion and ultimately provide the proof that something is indeed wrong or has become better.

Sometimes close is good enough

Another important point to those utilizing quality indicators is that "close does count". Quality indicators are not meant to be completely accurate, but to error on the side of false positives. As opposed to the rigors of science where accuracy and precision are required to reach conclusions, in quality, there may be times indeed where having a good idea of where things are may suffice enough to take action. In other words, sometimes close is good enough. The only caution here is that we need to be collectively aware of data bias. People who have an emotional or other type of investment in the outcome, may be too eager to accept or reject the outcome based more on their opinion rather than a comparative view of the data or by not listening to the consensus discussion amongst peers.

Blame the process not the person

The use of process analysis is not new, however it is quite fresh to the concepts of applying it to EMS performance information. Yet the concept is emphasized by so many healthcare quality organizations such as the Institute for Healthcare Improvement it is hard to ignore what they have been through and clearly concluded. It is true that 80-90% of all problems within a given industry are caused by flaws in the "system" rather than the people. This is not just folklore or hypothesis, it is a long standing – tried and true conclusion that everyone from Donald Berwick to Malcom Baldrige have lived through. It has been my experience that we administrators and evaluators especially in EMS have great difficulty with this paradigm shift. We are used to pointing fingers and holding "someone" accountable for the mistake. All the while never realizing that the mistake was made because system (we) failed to provide the information and tools necessary for that person to be successful. So we ask the person why did you make this mistake while instead we should be asking ourselves why did the mistake occur? Or where did this person go wrong? When we should be asking where the system (we) went wrong? You will find this theme of holding systems accountable over people throughout this textbook.

The Three Major Components of a
EMS Quality Improvement Program (QIP)

Whether the QIP is part of a large EMS system or a small ambulance organization, in its most basic terms, the concept of quality improvement is about changing the behavior of people or the parts of a certain activity with the goal of producing a better outcome. So the process of getting people to do something better is highly dependent on motivating them to do it.

Two things that help them to be motivated (other than paying them money) are to provide objective performance information that was put together by them and about them. The information serves the purpose of a map and shows them where they are now and helps them to pick a path for where they want to go. It is interesting to note that while applying the principles of evaluating data and motivating people to perform at higher levels is relatively new to EMS, it has been around for a long time and in fact has been very well demonstrated in our national pastime, namely the game of professional baseball. Nowhere else do you find such a clear and well executed example of people motivated to perform better based upon well-defined and trusted information.

"What is a system? A system is a network of interdependent components that work together to try to accomplish the aim of the system. A system must have an aim. Without an aim, there is no system. The aim of the system must be clear to everyone in the system, and include plans for the future. The aim is a value judgment.

"A system must be managed. It will not manage itself. Left to themselves in the Western world, components become selfish, competitive, independent profit centers, and thus destroy the system. The secret is cooperation between components toward the aim of the organization. We cannot afford the destructive effect of competition."

The Three Components
The following distinguishes the three components;
   1. System Evaluation
      EMS system evaluation is the collection of information in the form of patient care records, aggregate data and organizing that information into standardized reporting formats sometime called indicators or measures. The reports are then communicated to groups or teams of workers and users to determine the level of acceptable performance (benchmarks) and whether or not action to improve is needed.

   2. System Quality Improvement
      Quality improvement is the action side of the process. Once consensus is met regarding taking action, the action is transformed into a quality initiative where it is implemented, monitored, re-evaluated and sustained as necessary. This is often referred to in quality circles as the Plan-Do-Check-Act (PDCA) strategy for system improvement. The "check" portion of this process is highly dependent on the previous "system evaluation" component.

3. Patient Safety Events

Lastly, the patient safety component deals entirely with smaller and often individual performance or adverse events that need urgent or immediate attention and action. The character of this component is often looked at as the negative or punitive side of quality and though it is one of the major components of a comprehensive QI program, this is one of the important reasons why it is strongly recommended that we separate and draw this process out distinct of the other two components. Because good CQI requires the buy-in of the people who do the work, we should work very hard to have a positive attitude and encourage participation. However, a solid and comprehensive process for dealing with adverse patient safety events is imperative to both the overall function of QI and the health of our patients.

The three major components of a comprehensive EMS Quality Program

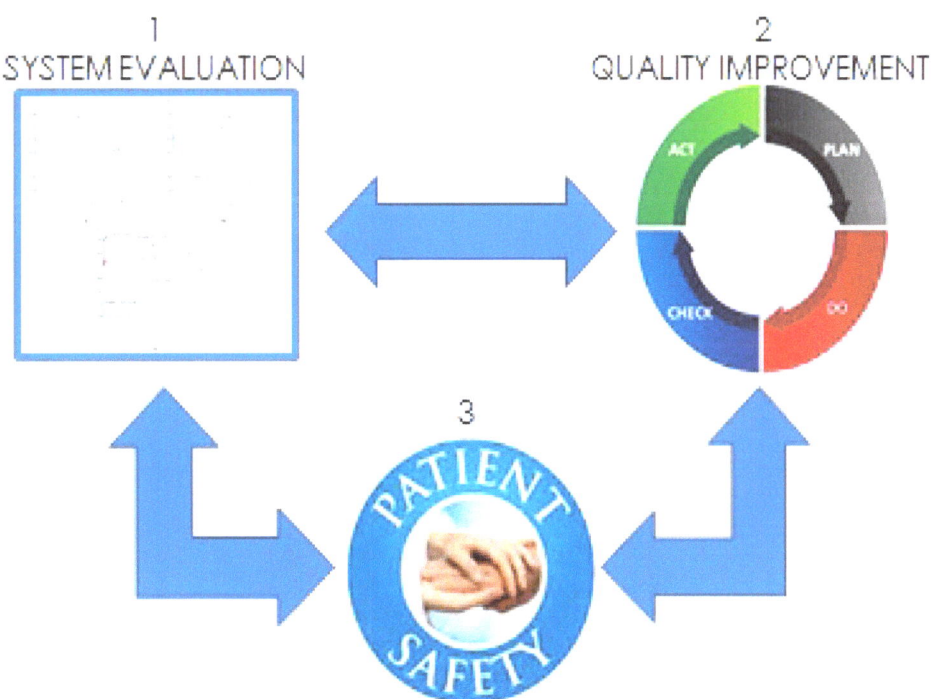

The First Component

EMS System Evaluation

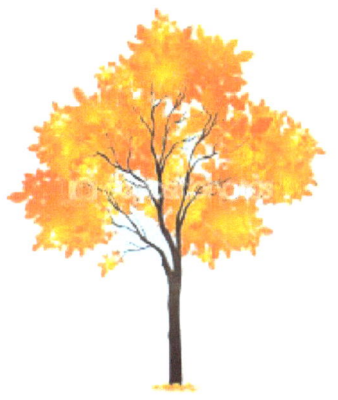

"Simplicity is the ultimate sophistication."
-Leonardo Davinci

Data Management 101

Understanding how data flows in an EMS system can often be daunting and over complicated. It doesn't have to be that way. For CQI mangers, simplicity should be the trump card. Information is information. The variables lie in how you captures and sort it out into usable and trusted information. Below is a diagram of how one EMS system manages quality information.

FLOW OF DATA INTO INFORMATION IN AN EMS SYSTEM

STAGE 1
EMS INFORMATION CAPTURED and STORED

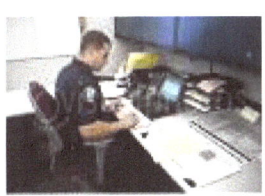

Data System	Data System	Data System Registries	Data System Registries
↓	↓	↓	↓
PROVIDER (A) PCR Record	PROVIDER (B) PCR Record	HOSPITAL (A) Pt Record	HOSPITAL (B) Pt Record

STAGE 2
INFORMATION DEFINED

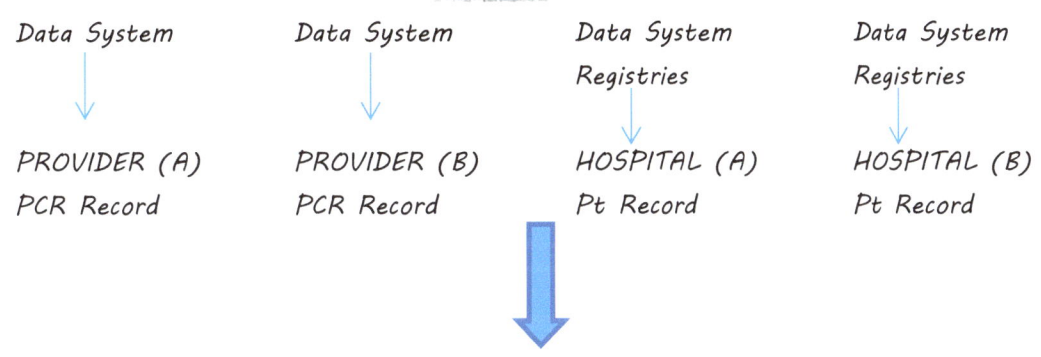

Performance Measure/Indicator Defined by Stakeholders	Performance Measure/Indicators Defined by Stakeholders	Performance Measure/Indicators Defined by Stakeholders	Performance Measure/Indicators Defined by Stakeholders

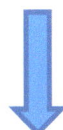

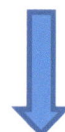

STAGE 3
INFORMATION REPORTED

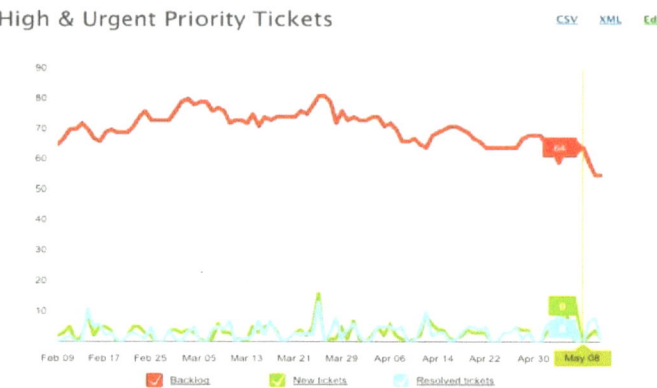

CQI Report	CQI Report	CQI Report	CQI Report
Generated	Generated	Generated	Generated
Reporting	Reporting	Reporting	Reporting
System	System	System	System

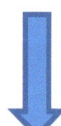

STAGE 4
INFORMATION EALUATED and ACTED ON
THROUGH CQI INITIATIVE

EMS CQI Team	EMS CQI Team	EMS CQI Team	EMS CQI Team
System Oversight	System Oversight	System Oversight	System Oversight
Committee	Committee	Committee	Committee

20

Keep it Simple, Stupid.

More often than not we have the tendency to complicate rather than simplify. We assume that sophistication equals results, brilliance, performance, and intelligence but it doesn't. More information, more choices, and more products are not better. In fact it is the exact opposite, more is actually less and can cause your colleagues and audience and especially EMS professionals to disengage.

EMS has activity and that activity is recorded at different points of a call and by different parties. Like most things in this world whether EMS or not, what happens at the beginning, sets the stage and effects the quality of everything that follows. To repeat the words of Paul Batalden, Medical Director, and Senior Fellow at the Institute for Healthcare Improvement (IHI); "every system is perfectly designed to get the results you get". More simply, if junk goes in, then you will most certainly get junk out at the other end. It's not the systems fault that it only has junk. Sometimes, the entire value of any body of data is completely dependent upon the quality of how well the event was documented and by whom.

EMS Documentation and the Patient Care Record (PCR)

It all begins at a beginning and the beginning in EMS is when the care provider whether EMT or paramedic initiates the PCR. This is also known as the key entry point of patient call documentation and data entry. Creating standards and regular training on appropriate techniques for both written and electronic patient care documentation is crucial to an accurate and trusted EMS information system. Unfortunately, this is an area that is often neglected by organizations. The results are poor and inconsistent quality reports.

Providing frequents and regularly scheduled training and updates on patient care documentation should be a priority for the CQI Program and an intense part of on-going training for the providers who document. Written standards, check sheets, drop downs and other default features should be sought out and made easily available as resources or checkpoints for patient care documenters. The providers should also have a clear understanding at least on an elementary level as to how the PCR is translated and converted to data and system CQI reports.

Having ownership and investing in the process will also enhance their performance and increase their motivation to be conscientious about their role in providing information. This part of collecting information in EMS systems continues to be an area that needs great attention and has a large capacity for improvement. In any system, the true experts in providing the best information are those at the front of the lines. EMS needs to provide a strong and vigorous support system for improving patient care documentation and sustaining quality in PCR standards.

Data Mining

Data mining is a term often used to describe the computational process of discovering patterns in large data sets. The goal of the data mining process is to extract information from a data set and transform it into an understandable structure for further use. Most EMS Quality Managers work with a data specialist or "data miner" to develop an analysis step which defines the goal of the data mine. For example, in EMS we may often use a tool known as an Indicator Specification Sheet (ISS). An ISS used to translate exactly what the question or/measure asking and exactly how it should be answered. All of the measures displayed in appendix #5 of this book are in the ISS format. A query or data mining exercise is translated and prepared by the data miner who is familiar with the data bank or system. The process involves data management aspects from developing a model and translating appropriate metrics, measures, indicators to the final reporting and post-processing of discovered information.

The process of data mining can be automatic or semi-automatic depending on types and quantities of data. Other types of extracts can be performed such as to extract previously unknown interesting patterns such as groups of data records (cluster analysis), unusual records (anomaly detection) and dependencies (association rule mining).

Other terms such as *data dredging*, *data fishing*, and *data snooping* refer to the use of data mining methods to sample parts of a larger population data set that are too small for reliable statistical evaluation. However, these methods can be used in creating new hypothesis to test against other larger data populations

Role of the Data Specialist

All QIP's should have dedicated personnel whose role it is to transform PCR information into a data base and then translate the data into larger aggregate reports. It is recommended that these staff personnel be separate and distinct in their role from those who manage and coordinate the QIP. This staff should also have basic working knowledge on the data system and how it functions within the operating systems within the organization. Troubleshooting, updating and washing data should be included in their job descriptions.

Making Your Data Simple

In general and for the purposes of dealing with people who work in EMS quality circles, "keep it simple" is a good philosophy. The following are simple recommendations when collecting and reporting data in a quality culture.

1. Pick the least amount of work for the evaluator.
2. Use the most essential information for decision making.
3. Reduce the amount of moving parts.
4. Choose the smallest and simplest words.
5. Use math only if essential.
6. Make the presentation as visually pleasing as possible.

Data Translation Sheet (DTS)

A typical Data Translation Sheet (DTS) is used to help data specialist within organizations understand specifically what data points and reporting criteria quality managers and their teams may want. Many times this sheet is completed by the data specialist who is either reviewing the Indicator Spec Sheet (ISS) or virtually face to face with the quality manager or designee who is seeking the information. Note: Enclosed in appendix (2) of this book is a copy of a typical Data Translation Sheet

Sources of data acquisition in EMS

Instead of naming specific proprietary examples of data collection systems, models and platforms currently used in EMS (most of you know who they are) I will focus more on the common sources and their most likely use in applying them to providing information to the EMS QI Manager.

Typical Sources for EMS systems

Structural Data: National & State Health Agencies, Census Bureau
Process Data: Provider Agencies, Dispatch Agencies, Patients
Outcome Data: Hospitals, Specialty Centers, Registries, Patients

Patient Registries

Patient registries are the future of EMS outcome information. With all of the difficulties getting "In-hospital" information that is critically important to "pre" hospital information, registries are a promising source of very difficult to obtain outcome information. Current registries such as the Cardiac Arrest Registry to Enhance Survival (CARES) and the California Stroke Registry are just two examples of places where solid outcome information is reported by hospitals and made available to EMS regulatory and provider agencies. Due to the complicated patient information laws and some reluctance on the part of hospitals to provide outcome information outside of their corporate structure, an increase in the utilization of data registries are more likely to become the primary source of aggregate outcome data for EMS systems. For these reasons, it is incumbent upon EMS systems to promote and support national and regional patient registries.

Data Warehousing

A data warehouse is a non-volatile time-variant repository of an organization's electronically stored data, designed to facilitate reporting and analysis. It is a copy of transaction data specifically structured for query and analysis. A Data warehouse is a subject-oriented, integrated, time-variant and non-volatile collection of data in support of management's decision making process"
This definition of the data warehouse focuses on data storage. However, the means to retrieve and analyze data, to extract, transform and load data, and to manage the data dictionary are also considered essential components of a data warehousing system. Many references to data warehousing use this broader context. Thus, an expanded definition for data warehousing includes business intelligence tools, tools to extract, transform and load data into the repository, and tools to manage and retrieve metadata.

Probabilistic Linkage

Currently there are times when we are connecting or cross-referencing two or more databases. This technique is called "Probabilistic linkage". This is when we search and find records in a data set that refer to the same entity but in different data sources (e.g., data files, books, websites, databases).

Abstracting and Annotating,

Of the other ways of obtaining good and reliable data, abstracting and annotating are most reliable but also the most time consuming. Often reserved more for research projects than quality programs, these techniques may need to be used if the information is not automatically collected by a data system or if the collection process is unreliable. Abstracting requires the quality manager to take away or "pick out" the most important data from a set of records.

Annotating

The process of annotating requires the quality manager to make observations and critical comments based upon documented activity. Both of these are labor-intensive, time consuming and often more related more to the "old school" quality improvement programs where page by page Patient care reports (PCR) reviews are the hallmark ways of finding the stuff you need to get "evidence" that things are wrong.

There is definitely a place for these two techniques of gathering data and I am not advocating throwing them out, but I do think there are better ways to find out what is going on in your system if getting the information close enough to make some decisions about what is going well and not so well. Interestingly enough, there are some new and really powerful innovations being made in the area of voice and narrative recognition software programs that may be the beginning of having the best of both worlds.

Narrative Recognition Software

There are great strides being made in the area of narrative recognition development especially in the software programs that are designed to detect and recognize common patterns of words or letters in the narrative of a patient document or care records and then to capture and record the specific words as data.

The Down Side of Data

- Concept of Reverse Engineering
- The perpetual "Data Imperative "don't understand/always need me/ time you get it- it will be obsolete

Pulling Out Information (Data)

The most common format for obtaining and reporting aw data is in the table format. On occasion, no further transformation of the data may be required. The concept of keeping things simple may work for the people who created the query or know the data well, but in most cases as with the data table shown below choosing an easier reporting format needs to be a consideration.

Example of Typical Data Reporting Table

Date	Transports	Response	Average
1/1/2012	5465	7176	6206.833
2/1/2012	5154	6731	6206.833
3/1/2012	5532	7257	6206.833
4/1/2012	5267	6896	6206.833
5/1/2012	5552	7235	6206.833
6/1/2012	5306	6989	6206.833
7/1/2012	5178	6864	6206.833

EMS Data Management

While Quality Managers should be encouraged to be involved in the management of the data system, it is NOT recommended that they take on the dual role of quality and Data System Managers. Instead of punching data entry keys, they should strive to be experts in asking the right questions of their data as well as interpreting and communicating the answers as objectively as possible.

With this scope in mind, it becomes incumbent of the Quality Manager to know that his purpose for the data system is to answer quality oriented questions rather than to understand how the data system operates and gathers information. It is best to leave the actual data queries and reporting to the data experts. After all, these are the people who are paid to understand and operate these systems and they are also an important checks and balance in the overall process.

The most important part of what a Quality Manager should know about his data system is how the data will be defined, collected and measured rather than how the machines store and retrieve the data. Quality Mangers should be more about letting "data people" know what it is they want and evaluating the results from a clinical, operational and purely quality point of view. In other words, telling the data system operators "this is what I want – make it happen." The rest should be the data people operating their magic. My observations have been that Quality Managers should be less into data driven systems and much more into "people" driven systems.

So, in fairness to our data people, we need to be clear what we want and how we want it done. So this is where the quality indicator becomes such an important tool. It is the tool that marries the data to the chart or table or any reporting format which in the end tells the story about what we have asked. Any good data systems operator will tell you that the results are only as good as the hypothesis. In other words, what goes in - comes out. If you ask for data in a crappy way, you will get a crappy result. It's not the data system operators fault, that is just the basic rule all data systems. They are all perfectly designed for you to get the perfect answer to whatever you ask. So you better ask the right question.

This is the most important value of utilizing a quality indicator. A quality indicator is the tool that you can use to reach consensus on what the clinicians, subject experts or other pertinent stakeholders want to ask as well as what the data operators need to know to obtain and produce the answers. The indicators provide what data operators call "operational definitions" which clearly defines the measure, the instrument to measure and the procedure for measuring. A good quality indicator has a well written and well defined explanation that has been agreed upon by all the stakeholders. In quality, the indicator is spelled out on an ISS. The ISS should have a section on it where the stakeholders are translating into a workable data sheet exactly what they want the data specialist to collect. At a minimum all of the following data collection questions need to be answered before the collection begins;

1. Who will collect the data?
2. Why are you collecting the data?
3. What methods will be used to collect it?
4. What specific data elements to be collected?
5. When will the data be collected?
6. Where will the data be collected?
7. How will the data be measured?
8. What format or medium will the data/measure be presented or reported?
9. What training is needed for the data collection?

Validity and Reliability
Validity refers to how well a test measures what it is purported to measure.
Why is it necessary? While reliability is necessary, it alone is not sufficient. For a test to be reliable, it also needs to be valid. For example, if your scale is off by 5 lbs., it reads your weight every day with an excess of 5lbs. The scale is reliable because it consistently reports the same weight every day, but it is not valid because it adds 5lbs to your true weight. It is not a valid measure of your weight.

Types of Validity
Face Validity ascertains that the measure appears to be assessing the intended construct under study. The stakeholders can easily assess face validity. Although this is not a very "scientific" type of validity, it may be an essential component in enlisting motivation of stakeholders. If the stakeholders do not believe the measure is an accurate assessment of the ability, they may become disengaged with the task. Example: If a measure of art appreciation is created all of the items should be related to the different components and types of art. If the questions are regarding historical time periods, with no reference to any artistic movement, stakeholders may not be motivated to give their best effort or invest in this measure because they do not believe it is a true assessment of art appreciation.

Construct Validity is used to ensure that the measure is actually measure what it is intended to measure (i.e. the construct), and not other variables. Using a panel of "experts" familiar with the construct is a way in which this type of validity can be assessed. The experts can examine the items and decide what that specific item is intended to measure. Students can be involved in this process to obtain their feedback.

Example: A women's studies program may design a cumulative assessment of learning throughout the major. The questions are written with complicated wording and phrasing. This can cause the test inadvertently becoming a test of reading comprehension, rather than a test of women's studies. It is important that the measure is actually assessing the intended construct, rather than an extraneous factor.

Criterion-Related Validity is used to predict future or current performance - it correlates test results with another criterion of interest. *Example*: If a physics program designed a measure to assess cumulative student learning throughout the major. The new measure could be correlated with a standardized measure of ability in this discipline, such as an ETS field test or the GRE subject test. The higher the correlation between the established measure and new measure, the more faith stakeholders can have in the new assessment tool.

Formative Validity when applied to outcomes assessment it is used to assess how well a measure is able to provide information to help improve the program under study. Example: When designing a rubric for history one could assess student's knowledge across the discipline. If the measure can provide information that students are lacking knowledge in a certain area, for instance the Civil Rights Movement, then that assessment tool is providing meaningful information that can be used to improve the course or program requirements.

Sampling Validity (similar to content validity) ensures that the measure covers the broad range of areas within the concept under study. Not everything can be covered, so items need to be sampled from all of the domains. This may need to be completed using a panel of "experts" to ensure that the content area is adequately sampled. Additionally, a panel can help limit "expert" bias (i.e. a test reflecting what an individual personally feels are the most important or relevant areas.

Example: When designing an assessment of learning in the theatre department, it would not be sufficient to only cover issues related to acting. Other areas of theatre such as lighting, sound, functions of stage managers should all be included. The assessment should reflect the content area in its entirety.

What are some ways to improve validity?
1. Make sure your goals and objectives are clearly defined and operationalized. Expectations of students should be written down.
2. Match your assessment measure to your goals and objectives. Additionally, have the test reviewed by faculty at other schools to obtain feedback from an outside party who is less invested in the instrument.
3. Get students involved; have the students look over the assessment for troublesome wording, or other difficulties.
4. If possible, compare your measure with other measures, or data that may be available.

Reliability and the Types of Reliability:

Reliability is the degree to which an assessment tool produces stable and consistent results.

Test-retest reliability is a measure of reliability obtained by administering the same test twice over a period of time to a group of individuals. The scores from Time 1 and Time 2 can then be correlated in order to evaluate the test for stability over time.

Example: A test designed to assess student learning in psychology could be given to a group of students twice, with the second administration perhaps coming a week after the first. The obtained correlation coefficient would indicate the stability of the scores.

Parallel forms reliability is a measure of reliability obtained by administering different versions of an assessment tool (both versions must contain items that probe the same construct, skill, knowledge base, etc.) to the same group of individuals. The scores from the two versions can then be correlated in order to evaluate the consistency of results across alternate versions.

Example: If you wanted to evaluate the reliability of a critical thinking assessment, you might create a large set of items that all pertain to critical thinking and then randomly split the questions up into two sets, which would represent the parallel forms.

Inter-Rater Reliability
Inter-rater reliability is a measure of reliability used to assess the degree to which different judges or raters agree in their assessment decisions. Inter-rater reliability is useful because human observers will not necessarily interpret answers the same way; raters may disagree as to how well certain responses or material demonstrate knowledge of the construct or skill being assessed.

Example: Inter-rater reliability might be employed when different judges are evaluating the degree to which art portfolios meet certain standards. Inter-rater reliability is especially useful when judgments can be considered relatively subjective. Thus, the use of this type of reliability would probably be more likely when evaluating artwork as opposed to math problems.

Internal consistency reliability is a measure of reliability used to evaluate the degree to which different test items that probe the same construct produce similar results.

Average inter-item correlation is a subtype of internal consistency reliability. It is obtained by taking all of the items on a test that probe the same construct (e.g., reading comprehension), determining the correlation coefficient for each *pair* of items, and finally taking the average of all of these correlation coefficients. This final step yields the average inter-item correlation.

Split-half reliability is another subtype of internal consistency reliability. The process of obtaining split-half reliability is begun by "splitting in half" all items of a test that are intended to probe the same area of knowledge (e.g., World War II) in order to form two "sets" of items. The *entire* test is administered to a group of individuals, the total score for each "set" is computed, and finally the split-half reliability is obtained by determining the correlation between the two totals "set" scores.

The Concept of Reverse Engineering

Indicators also help to determine what a data system should look like prior to actually spending the money to develop one. The concept of reverse engineering is where a data system designer actually asks the questions to be answered by the data system BEFORE it is actually built - a rather novel concept which you would think should be widespread, but not so as I have learned. In many cases, data systems developed at enormous costs and the designing of such systems were primarily done by who else, but the data specialists and technical experts who had no idea what the system was really supposed to do.[20] [26] It's not their fault. Most of the time they built what the users wanted - a data system with little forethought as to the purpose of the data. Consequently, EMS has many data systems today that produce information that often has little or no value to the end users. Indicators can work against this problem by being an integral part of the original design of a data system. By first asking the questions of stakeholders and end users, the answers can be defined and consensus can be reached as to the purpose of the data. Then once all the indicators are established, the data can now be determined and defined to produce the data.

Some Final Recommendations Regarding Data Management

I realize we may be swimming upstream, but I really don't understand why the regulatory and coordination central EMS agencies are in the data business. My recommendations to all EMS regulatory agencies or any agency that manages several providers and agencies, is to **NOT** get into the data management business or if you are already in it – get out as fast as you can EMS agencies should be quality mangers not data managers. Doing so just gives everyone who should be responsible for providing reliable information (data) someone to blame when things don't work. Data system proprietors love the fact that everyone works independent of each other and having their own way of providing data and then trying mix it all together at the system level. This just creates an endless vacuum of problems that need fixing and by the time most systems figure out what is wrong, it's time to purchase a new system with all the new innovations. Agencies that mange large or multi-provider systems should simply define what reports they want and then make it incumbent on their providers to provide "finished reports" that answer quality indicators pre-defined by the community they serve. Nothing sexy or powerful – just reliable and valid. In other words don't send me a disc full of dispatch data, send me the final report which shows your 90th percentile response times for last quarter. This is a novel concept. Yes, I mean make THEM accountable for having reliable and consistent data. Send someone out every 3-6 months to sample their data and verify what they are sending you, but please, please, EMS agencies need to get out of the data business. Be the central depository for accurate and accountable quality information, not the place they blame when their data is not valid or the results of you crunching their data is that it looks like crap.

Quality Indicators & Measures

<u>General Description</u>

"Quality Indicators, which are sometimes called measures, metrics, benchmarks, as well as other terms depending upon the nature of their use, are the "growl of the Sabertooth." They are the signal which stimulates us and tell us whether we should get up and run or simply go back to sleep.

<u>The Quality Indicator: The Most Powerful Consensus Tool</u>

In the world of quality improvement, indicators are your "go-to" tool for building consensus and trust of your information within a CQI constituent group. [19] An important objective in the CQI process is trying to eliminate as much controversy and mistrust as possible. This is not always an easy task considering the host of aggressive personalities that EMS tends to attract as a profession. It is often said in quality circles that "he who has the data is king" and I strongly agree. But there are conditions to my agreement. First, it is critical that all the data is collected in a way and from a source that has been previously agreed upon by the group. If this condition is satisfied and the data is considered to be trustworthy by the group, then I have seen with my own eyes the almost complete elimination of subjective controversy and innuendo that can be slung around a room from one person to another without regard to what is the truth. The nice thing is we're pretty good at collecting data and throwing the money at it. The problem we often run into is even with good data we sometimes don't know how to communicate it to the group. This is where quality indicators become so important to the CQI process.

Organizing the data in a pre-determined and agreed upon format (quality indicators) takes away a lot of the problems inherent to a CQI group decision making process. While it seems to be impossible to eliminate controversy completely from a process, using indicators to show the data puts the information in a very objective format and tends to remove subjectivity, barriers and controversy. Quality indicators are the core method for communicating your data and should be the core tools of any EMS CQI program.

<u>What are Quality Indicators?</u>

Quality indicators are the tools that define the data, communicate the information, establish the consensus, stimulate the discussion and ultimately provide the proof that something is indeed better. Simply, CQI is heavily dependent on motivating people to be better just like the coaches of a sports team, quality indicators are the key tools that coaches use to motivate change and improvement. It makes no difference what EMS culture you work within, whether a hospital, or the rank and file of a fire department, or in the management structure of a patient transportation industry or whether you choose traditional PDCA, Six Sigma, Lean, or Rapid Cycle Improvement as your model for CQI. It all comes down to communication and motivation and it is the quality indicator that provides the primary tool and language for accomplishing this ultimate goal. Quality Indicators are the guts of any well performing CQI program. Quality Indicators are tools that are shaped and formed by those who use them. Often called quality measures, quality metrics, quality benchmarks, quality indicators can mean many things to many people. But for our purposes and in the simplest terms quality indicators are "gauges" that give us some idea of how our systems are doing. Just as a fuel gauge on a car tells us how we are doing on fuel or in the case of the American economy, the Dow Jones Industrials indicate how the stock market is performing at a given moment in time.

A single quality indicator may contain one or many of the most important parts (activities and outcomes) of our system held together and displayed in an easy to read format that instantaneously tells us how the majority of these parts are performing. So the first requirement of a quality indicator is that it must contain value that communicates efficiently, "This is how we are doing".

There is a very important second part of a quality indicator which is determining consensus definition. That is to say that a quality indicator must also have a generally accepted meaning that all the users trust and which says the same thing in the same way to all those who use it. In order for a quality indicator to function, it must have been previously defined and agreed to by its users. This is called consensus definition. Just as when we measure the pulse of a patient whose rate is below 40 beats per minute (bpm), the pulse rate alone has little value to the clinician unless it can be put together with a patient that can be seen, touched and heard. In this case the indicator (pulse less than 40 bpm) must have a person for us to see so that we can define whether the rate is good or bad. In the case of a patient who is a triathlon athlete and who is fully alert with normal skin signs and in no apparent distress, this is perhaps a good pulse rate. In much the same way, for us to truly understand and digest a quality indicator, we must define what it will mean first. An indicator must be defined prospectively by the users as to specifically what question will it answer and how the answer will be communicated. Therefore, it is paramount that all indicators start with a question that is agreed upon by all users through consensus. What do you want to know? How will it be answered? To answer these important questions, the indicator needs to be captured and recorded on what we call an indicator specification sheet, or what is abbreviated as a "spec sheet" or "ISS".

Structure, Process and Outcome
In most EMS systems, it is best to organize system information into three primary attributes (structure, process and outcome). (5) (6) (11)

The attributes-components of this system are expressed through quality indicators. These indicators are your tools for interpreting and communicating the need for change. This change is effected by pressures brought about by the collegial review and thoughtful decisions of the stakeholders within the system.

In most cases, the change creates the pressures within the system to effect the change that hopefully in the end provides the inspired improvement in the outcome measures of our services in most cases. These attributes create the cause and the effect relationship within all quality systems, and accordingly apply as well and in the same way to the formal CQI circles where we EMS CQI managers live and breathe. Together, these components make up the "great equation" that further defines the formal foundation for evaluating our systems by the use of quality indicators. For the purpose of illustration, we shall review the characteristics of the three types of quality attributes, which make up our system of evaluation, and also look at the relationship they have with one another as expressed in "the great equation". That equation is made up of the "things" in a system, what they do, or the "activities" within the system and when combined together, what outcomes do they produce?

Structure + Process = Outcome

EMS System Things + EMS System Activities = EMS System Effects

An even more specific way of saying this would be: People + Defibrillations = Cardiac Arrest Saves. In this case, the defibrillators are the "things" or structural attributes. The delivery of defibrillations is the "activity" or the process indicator and the cardiac arrest saves would be the result or the "effect". So putting it into CQI terms: the structures and process create the outcome.

Structural Indicators (Things)
Structural Indicators are things within a system, i.e. number of ambulances per patient population, number of hospitals with STEMI services, number of paramedics per response unit, number of trauma centers, etc. For example, there are 27 Advanced Life Support Units available to respond to emergencies in the EMS system.

Process Indicators (Activities)
These are activities or procedures that happen within a given system. For example; response times under eight minutes, proportion of cardiac arrest patients who receive defibrillations, IV starts, etc. Processes are often broken down into steps. For example, steps in the process of dispatching an ambulance would be: 1) 911 Call initiated; 2) 911 Call received; 3) Ambulance dispatched, etc.

Outcome Indicators (Effects)
By far the most important of the three types of indicators, outcome is where and what we are ultimately trying to improve. Outcome indicators are the actual results things have on the system based upon their respective activities or actions within the system. For example, it is a well-accepted theory that cardiac save rates (outcomes) are dependent upon the number of defibrillators (structures) available and how readily they are deployed (processes). One would conclude based upon solid science available in the literature, that the slower a EMS system responds with defibrillators to a cardiac arrest event, the lower the save rate and visa versa. Other outcome measures would be: hospitals stay times, morbidity rates, mortality rates, etc. Obviously, the structures and processes in a system make up our "cause" in the analysis, while the outcome is the "effect". When we put it all together, we can see that the components are related to one another proportionally and can be expressed as an equation:

Structure (things) + Processes (activities) = Outcome (effect)
When we place numeric values to represent each of these components as illustrated above in our examples, we have transformed the components from an attribute to a quality indicator which can be quantified and qualified. Hence, it follows that these components are most often described numerically in the form of structure, process and outcome quality indicators. Using the indicator as our values, we call this expression the "great equation" because it clearly and concisely communicates both what and how we look at in our systems. It tells the story that things are done in a system that have a cumulative effect and, like all great equations, one side directly affects the other. For example, by increasing the number of AEDs (structures) available in the system, we theoretically should improve the process (number of patients defibrillated) and that should have a cumulative-positive effect on the number of cardiac arrest survivors (outcomes).

The inverse is theoretically true as well. While all parts of the equation are important, a final point should be made about the proper interpretation of this equation. That is in all cases, we are most interested in making the outcome or the "end product" the primary focus of what we are really trying to improve. This is to say that while it is noble and most heartwarming to have an improved process such as increased intubation success rate, this attribute is meaningless if we are not improving the outcomes of those patients who need intubation in general.

Classifying EMS System Quality Indicators based upon Frequency and type of Use

The use of quality indicators can be further organized and categorized by their particular importance and the frequency of their use within a system. The three major categories of indicators defined in this manner are: Core, Tertiary and Adhoc.

Core Indicators are chosen indicators within a system which tell a story of how well a system is doing overall at a glance. They are truly the "Dow Jones Industrials" of your EMS system. Just as the Dow Jones Industrials are the primary indicators of the New York Stock Exchange, Core Indicators within an EMS System should quickly answer the question, how is my system performing overall? In EMS systems, Core indicators tend to look at the most important primarily components such as cardiac arrest, trauma, stroke, base hospital, STEMI and system utilization. Core indicators such as those displayed below should be published regularly and should be open and available to the public to review and comment.

Tertiary Indicators are measures that should be at the fingertips because they indicate important performance information but do not necessarily need to be reported or published on a regular basis. Tertiary Indicators may be indicators that are looking more closely at a part or "component" of a core or outcome indicator. For example, save rates of an EMS System may be a core indicator and the time to defibrillation may be tertiary as well as a process which has an effect on the core.

Adhoc Indicators are indicators that are developed at will or at the discretion of the CQI program. They may be long term or short term. They may be structural, process, or outcome depending on objective. An example of Adhoc Indicators may be the development of an indicator that measures pediatric drug errors for a one year period. Once the information has been gathered, studied and acted upon, can then be discarded or used again as needed. Often Adhoc Indicators are used for special projects or immediate or temporary concerns of a CQI group regarding their system.

Bi-variable, Single-variable and Continuous-Variable Indicators

Finally, indicators can also be classified by the way the data is collected and measured. For example, if the indicator end result is in percent (%), then that requires two pieces of data: first, the data for the numerator (small population) and then secondly, the data for the denominator (the larger population. Both of these portions of the data are required to perform the calculation to determine the final value of percent (%). One data value (numerator) is divided by the other value (denominator) to determine a percentage (%). Because we need **two values,** to get the final reporting value; this is called a **bi-variable** indicator. If you were measuring only one thing such as the number of cars in a parking lot, then this would be a single variable indicator. There is no need for a numerator in a single-variable.

The third type is called a "continuous" variable which is where we are dealing with data from measurements that can go on forever such as time, length, etc. Because they are continuous, we usually put this type of data into a bell shaped curve and look to determine a percentile such as the 90th or 80th. Response time compliance is commonly reported this way. In this example, a continuous variable may be reported as the ambulance is on scene within 7 mins 90% of the time.

In the same way, different types of indicators require different types of indicator spec sheets to match up with the type of indicator we plan to develop. In EMS, we most often use a bi-variable and percent (%) as our reporting value. But when we are measuring things like response or on scene time then we like to use continuous and look at the 90th percentile as a standard. Accordingly, when we use a single variable, we are looking at just one thing and these are usually structural indicators such as the number of certified EMTs or number of ambulances.

Appendix ( ) shows examples of fully completed Indicator Specification Sheets and a detailed step by step process for following the recommended three steps of indicator development.

Importance of consensus
Consensus driven by evidence based outcomes
"In God we trust; all others must bring data."
From the book, The Elements of Statistical Learning

Consensus in Decision Making
Organizing and clearly communicating important information about data is the key to facilitating a good decision on the part of the users. Quality indicators are used to interpret information and help make decisions. As previously discussed, quality indicators are only a tool. People make decisions, not data and not indicators. An indicator helps a group of people to look at information and interpret what it means, and/or to decide if the subject of the indicator requires something to be done to make it better.

Without the people, the quality indicator has no value and no meaning; on the other hand, a quality indicator is built and lives off of those who gave it birth and defined it. Evaluation is a process. Deciding what's important and what can make it better can be difficult if you are not organized in the approach.

Statistical Analysis for Quality Managers
"Numbers are Our Friends"

Honestly, do we really need to be that complicated? Sometimes we put things in such complicated terms that the only people who understand them are those who wrote them. The same is generally true in applying statistical analysis to quality information. It is my strong opinion that Quality Managers need to be much more concerned about what statistical measurements mean rather than how they were designed and the details of how the numbers were crunched.

So again, some simple rules help us out. Now days even statisticians would agree, the number crunching is more about software programing and coding than doing mathematical formulas. So for EMS Quality Mangers, it's much more important to be able to know what a statistical measurement is telling you about your system rather than the numerical definition or the formula for determining the measure. In other words, just put in the numbers and push the button and read the results. That's really all you need to know.

What Matters?
In general only five things really matter when evaluating 90% of our charts and measures;
1. Sample size,
2. Measurements about the averages or middle values,
3. Measurements spread out around the average or middle values
4. Percentiles,
5. Trends or how a things change over time?

Sampling: (The Rule of Thirty n=30)
In general, when sampling a data source - the larger your sample size, the more accurate your statistical measurements. However, when dealing with quality we again fall upon the concept that in most cases having a good idea of where you stand is just as valuable for decision making as to have the most rigorous mathematical and scientific results. Especially since we as quality mangers mostly limit our statistical queries to measurements to normal bell curve distributions and attributes of central tendency. In other words, we are not statisticians; we are quality mangers and should have strong understandings of what statistical measurements mean but not necessarily the theory and practical concepts of how they are determined. Accordingly, in the world of quality it is common for Quality Managers to trust a minimum sampling rule of at least thirty (30). My experience has been that for our simple measurements, I have seen minuscule differences when I used 30 data points vs. 500 data points. On the other hand, I have seen significant variations in sample sizes less than 30.

In many cases, statisticians will argue that there is no proof to the theory of the sampling rule of 30. Although I would argue that for our short and simple statistical measurements, fast is good and easy is even better. So I would recommend that if you are planning to submit your data to some statistical measurements - then all you need is at least 30 data points to be reasonably accurate. In most cases a quality measure/indicator spec sheet will identify the minimum sampling size required.

Rate vs. Sentinel

Rate: The number sample per entire population or samples over time is often called the "rate" of sampling. For example, if an inspector was examining the quality of apples passing by on a moving belt by randomly choosing one apple every 10 seconds, then this would be considered 1/10 sampling rate based upon time. Conversely, if the inspector was choosing 1 apple for every 10 that passed, then again this would be a rate of population. In both cases, the inspector is using a 10% sampling rate. So in the case of EMS service providers, determining a rate of sampling may be a more efficient way to monitor a quality indicator that has a high frequency/ low risk to the system.

Sentinel: The 100% measurement of a particular quality indicator or process is termed a sentinel event or indicator. In this case all (100%) of the apples on the belt are inspected for quality. Use of a sentinel rate for sampling may be indicated for low frequency/high risk activities within a system. In most cases a quality measure/indicator spec sheet will identify the rate of sampling or whether it is sentinel in the sampling.

Measurements around the Average or Middle Values. (Central Tendency)

Referred to by statisticians as measure of central tendency, these are single values that attempt to describe a set of data by identifying the central position within that set of data. They are also classed as summary statistics. The mean (often called the average) is most likely the measure of central tendency that you are most familiar with, but there are others, such as the median and the mode.

Mean

The mean (or average) is the most popular and well known measure of central tendency
Mean = sum of all values divided by total number of values

Median

The median is the middle score for a set of data that has been arranged in order of magnitude. Median = middle value when data arranged in numeric rank order

Mode

The mode is the most frequent score in our data set. On a histogram it represents the highest bar in a bar chart or histogram.
Mode = most common (repeated) value

Measures spread out around the Average or Middle values (Dispersed)

Dispersion (also called variability, scatter, or spread) shows how stretched out or squeezed a data sample is distributed around the average or middle of those values. The most common examples of measures of statistical dispersion are the variance, standard deviation and the range.

Variance

Variance is used as a measure of how far a set of numbers are spread out from the center or mean.

Standard Deviation

Standard deviation is a measurement which shows how widely spread (dispersed) the data is around the mean. The Standard Deviation is the "mean of mean". Basically, it is the square-root of the Variance (the mean of the differences between the data points and the average.

Range
The range is the spread between the highest and lowest data points. Also defined mathematically as the maximum data value minus the minimum data value.

Percentiles
Percentiles are defined as the portion of a whole. Most percentiles can be determined by multiplying by 100 to determine the percentile (%). What is tricky in EMS is when we are looking at continuous data such as time and want to determine a specific percentile (90%) of a group of data points. In this case we would rank the data ascending order. Then count the number of data points and then multiply by .90. The resulting answer will give you the number that represents the 90th % of all the data. In other words 90% of the data falls below this number.

Process Control Analysis
How Things Change Over Time

A process can be defined as a group of smaller tasks performed each day to bring about an end result such as registering patients, identifying needed health services, refilling prescriptions, ordering tests, etc. An example of interrelated systems would be in the physician office, where they provide multiple processes that are interrelated and considered the system. Furthermore, a physician's office may be one of many offices owned by a health care organization, and in this circumstance would be considered a system within a system.

Process Variation
Process variation occurs in all processes, and no process functions exactly the same way over time. How do we meet the demands for accountability and improvement when processes always vary? First we must understand variation.

Random or Common Cause is intrinsic to the process itself. It is the naturally occurring "noise" of the process. An example of common cause: the patient/resident response to medication will always vary within a group of patients/residents and even for one patient/resident over time.
Common causes refer to situations that are usually within care systems and processes (within the normal bell-shaped curve) that are ongoing, chronic, and persistent. These common causes may contribute to what is considered to be a "normal range of variation" within a process. The goal of quality improvement is not to eliminate, but to reduce variation in a process enough to produce and sustain stability. Common causes may also contribute to what are considered to be the less than desirable parts of a process.

Usually finding and resolving common causes of problems or variation is more time-consuming and may be more difficult for departments, services, and QI teams. The resolution of common causes of problems is important to continuous, incremental improvement of quality of care and services.

More on Process Control

Here is some wisdom from Dr. Donald Berwick Director of the Institute for Healthcare Improvement -- from almost 20 years ago,

"Plotting measurements over time it turns out, in my view, to be one of the most powerful devices we have for systemic learning...Several important things happen when you plot data over time. First, you have to ask what data to plot. In the exploration of the answer you begin to clarify aims, and also to see the system from a wider viewpoint. Where are the data? What do they mean? To whom? Who should see them? Why? These are questions that integrate and clarify aims and systems all at once.

Second, you get a leg up on improvement. When important indicators are continuously monitored, it becomes easier and easier to study the effects of innovation in real time, without deadening delays for setting up measurement systems or obsessive collections during baseline periods of inaction. Tests of change get simpler to interpret when we use time as a teacher...So convinced am I of the power of this principle of tracking over time that I would suggest this: If you follow only one piece of advice from this lecture when you get home, pick a measurement you care about and begin to plot it regularly over time. You won't be sorry."
[Berwick's 1995 Institute for Healthcare Improvement Forum plenary speech "Run to Space"]

Step by Step Using Process Control Charting Programs

We evaluate the data by using graphic representations of activities which show trends and variations over time.
1. Numerical soundness; Numbers match what you put in
2. Data Reliability; 90% of first result abnormalities is data related.
3. Look for mean and average; Mean is average
4. Common or Special causation; Statistical significance not absolute problem.
5. Trending; the seven tests

Trending

The process of showing by plot or process control chart, the upward, downward or level movement of an activity over a specified period of time.
Gestalt: Initial "gut" impression and instinctive or intuitive reactions to the overall view of a chart or table just in off the press is often times accurate assessment.

Statistically Significant

Statistical significance refers to whether any differences are observed between data groups being studied or whether they are real or whether due to chance. It's easy for non-scientists to misunderstand the term significant. To most EMS personnel, it means "important." But when researchers say the findings of a study were "statistically significant," they do not necessarily mean the findings are important. So the use of the term statistically significant particularly in quality circles means that it has met the statistical and mathematical qualifications to be consider two subjects to be different but the decision about whether that statistical difference is important or relevant to the quality of the system remains a deliberation and decision on the part of the subject experts and system stakeholders who own the process.

Process Variation: Common Cause: Variances within the lines

Special cause is extrinsic to the process and related to identifiable patient/resident or clinical characteristics, idiosyncratic practice patterns, or other factors that can be tracked or assigned to root causes. Special causes refer to sentinel events, one-time occurrences, or other unique, out of-the-ordinary circumstances that give rise to a variation from what are normally expected. Special causes account for what are called "outliers" – problems that happen in the "tails" of a normal, bell-shaped curve representing a particular process.

Case review and root cause analysis are needed to identify special cause and take action. Such variations, if negative (referred to as a Sentinel Event), can be quickly changed, and eliminated. Positive variations can be analyzed for replication as better or best practice.

Special Cause:
Possible source that causes a fundamental change in a process. Special cause variation signals a change in a process and can usually be traced back to a single source.

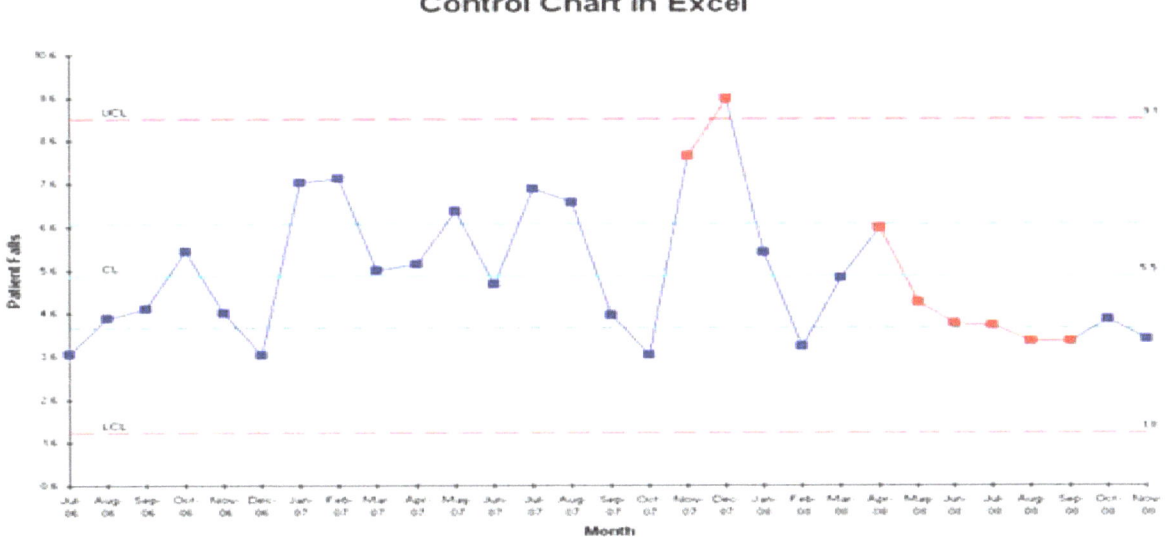

Control Chart in Excel

- *"Special Causes and Common Causes"*: Deming considered anomalies in quality to be variations outside the control limits of a process. Such variations could be attributed to one-time events called "special causes" or to repeated events called "common causes" that hinder quality.

- *Acceptable Defects*: Rather than waste efforts on zero-defect goals, Deming stressed the importance of establishing a level of variation, or anomalies, acceptable to the recipient (or customer) in the next phase of a process. Often, some defects are quite acceptable, and efforts to remove all defects would be an excessive waste of time and money

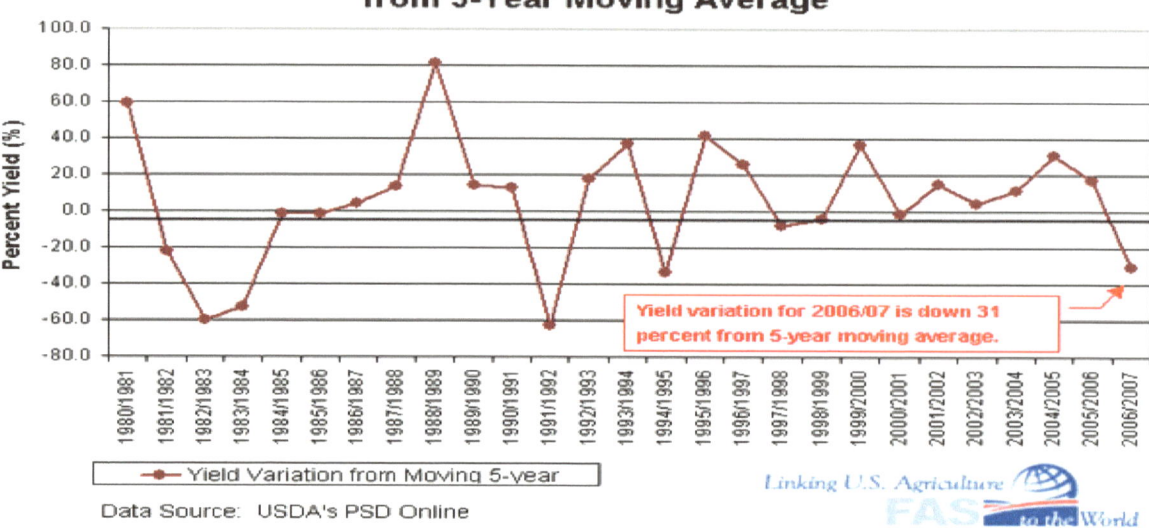

South Africa's Corn Yield Variation from 5-Year Moving Average

Yield variation for 2006/07 is down 31 percent from 5-year moving average.

Yield Variation from Moving 5-year

Data Source: USDA's PSD Online

Linking U.S. Agriculture FAS to the World

Statistics? We Don't Need No Stinking Statistics

In my experience in doing quality services in EMS for well over 25 years, one of the things that tends to discourage colleagues at the beginning, is the idea that to be a good quality manger, you should also be good at math to understand statistics. Let me just say that I have found this to be very untrue. What you do need is a good understanding of what the numbers mean to you and your constituent groups around the subject of quality. The skills of being a facilitator and consensus builder are far more valuable than be well versed at crunching numbers. I would also say that with today's software programs, it is a waste of valuable time for a quality manger to be doing the math. They should instead be simply pushing the buttons on their computers to have the software programs do the math. There are currently some very good programs for basic statistical analysis and process charting. Below are just a few;

Commercial Programs for Process Control Charting and Statistical analysis

There are several commercial types of software programs available that can easily be loaded onto windows operated PCS. They range from free to very expensive and from simple to fairly complex. Of course my recommendation is get the simplest one for the least costs.

IBM Programs; BP Charts

BP charts is a common process charting program that was developed and distributed as a free program. It is a very intuitive Microsoft-excel based program that allows you to simply input the data and press the button. Up pops a printable run chart or process chart like the one shown above - along with all of the statistical values already calculated and displayed.

QI Macros Software for PC's

Excel based software for performing control charts, histograms, Pareto & other statistical or CQI oriented charts. It also has some built-in data proofing and wizards to simplify analysis.

Other popular software

Similar programs can be reviewed at the following links; http://www.capterra.com/spc-software/ or by visiting our website@www.cemspi.org

Benchmarking and Best Practices

Benchmarking is the process of comparing processes and performance measures to bests or best practices from other companies. Dimensions typically measured are quality, time and cost. In the process of best practice benchmarking, administration identifies the best examples of EMS practices or similar healthcare practices and compares the results and processes. Benchmarking is used to measure performance using a specific indicator (cost per unit of measure, save rate, etc) resulting in a measure/indicator of performance that is then compared to others. Also referred to as "best practice benchmarks" or "process benchmarking," EMS is a relatively young industry in comparison to other industries and performance measures that could be considered "best practices" are not plentiful. In some circumstances, there may not be a best practice or benchmark for a system to compare itself. In this case, the community reaches consensus with input from the users, stakeholders and subject experts as to the details and standards of the benchmark.

Communicating with Charts

Ok, so you have some good information. You collected it from a reliable source and have validated its utility. You have also put it into an indicator spec sheet and obtained consensus on what the information will say. Now it is time to put the information into a format that makes it say what it is supposed to say in the easiest and most efficient way possible. Selecting the medium and format for presenting your information becomes just as important as what it says. Taking the time to prepare well cannot be overstated. This step in the process becomes what most people don't know about successful acting and teaching. Ninety percent of the execution of a good product is preparation. Taking the time to thoughtfully determine what the presentation needs to say and how you will say it is critical to the utility of a quality indicator.

Generally there are 3 main types of data analysis are needed for everyday business decisions - comparison, transition and composition of data.
So the first question to ask yourself is;
What do I want to show?
How the information compares?
What it is composed of?
How it is distributed?
How it relates to another variable?

Once you have decided these attributes of your presentation, consult the alga rhythm on appendix 2 of this textbook. This diagram can assist you to easily select the most appropriate chart for you presentation

Important considerations when making a presentation is to know your audience. Knowing your audience is a valuable part of preparing the presentation. These types of decisions are best served when the presenter has some background in basic learning theory such as the left brain vs. right brain learning theory often taught to professional educators.

Adult Learning Theory

Those who have formal teacher/instructor training tend to understand the group leadership dynamics better if you have been trained on some of the adult learning theories that can be applied to presenting and facilitating decision-making in groups. The concepts of left brain and right brain learning are particularly helpful when presenting. The short version of this learning theory says that adults absorb information which is complex or otherwise by two different pathways to the cerebral cortex. One if called the left brain which is said to be logical, technical, and sequential whereas the right brain likes to see and touch things with pictures and color. Most people are both but usually dominate in one or the other. A good test to determine which dominance is to ask a person which method of driving directions they would prefer;

1. The left brain dominance; this is where they prefer directions where a map is drawn out with colored lines and small colored cars showing direction or streets to turn.

or

2. Do they prefer a right brain dominant list of directions written out with sequential steps such as; 1. Turn left at Walnut Street; 2. Go two blocks and turn right, etc.

Presenting important information in both left and right brain ways helps your group to understand more clearly the information you are facilitating forth to help them make decisions. Using both charts and graphs both on a screen and in a handout as well as providing a table or other left brain set of black and white numbers showing the same information may very well help your mission of getting them to trust and understand the information and reach consensus quickly with less explanation.

Presenting

In many cases, it is good to hand-out the information in left brain written format showing details and definitions and then to follow with right brain pictures and color graphs on an overhead or power point projection. As a rule of thumb, the following is a quick guide to choosing an appropriate chart for a presentation of information before a group or committee.

- Structures (things) - usually are best represented by bar or pie graphs
- Processes (activities) - are almost always best to show over time in in line graph. *My favorites are process charts or run charts*
- *Outcomes (end results)- work best usually in a bar or column graph.*

Again, it is also very important to state and revisit the mission and purpose of the group review of each indicator chart. Thus, prior to presenting the objectives of the review and indicator could be presented or read in a question format.

EMS Quality Improvement

**Unlocking the Universal
PDCA model**

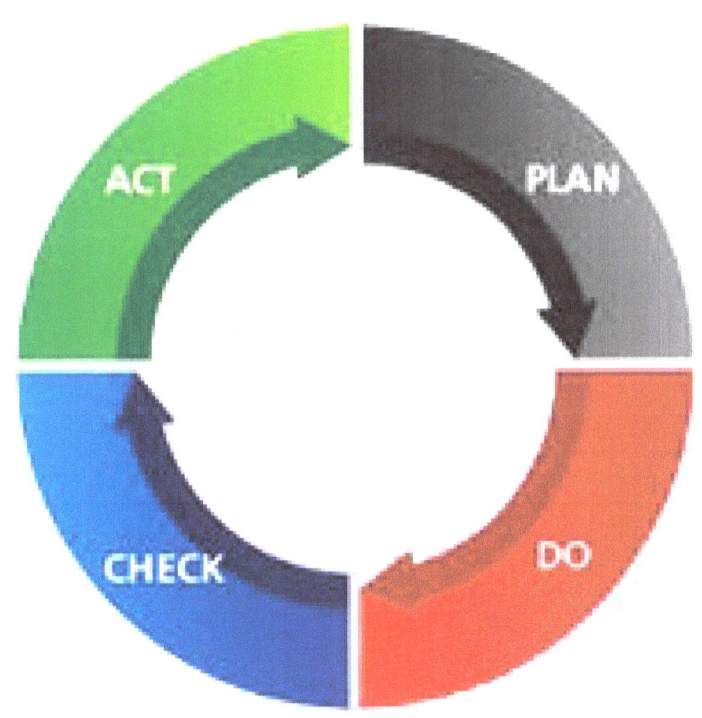

The Deming Cycle or Shewhart Cycle

Continuous Quality Improvement
The Universal PDCA Model

As a repetitive process to determine the next action, the Deming Cycle describes a simple method to test information before making a major decision. The 4 steps in the Deming Cycle are: Plan-Do-Check-Act (PDCA), also known as Plan-Do-Study-Act or PDSA. Deming called the cycle the *Shewhart Cycle*, after <u>Walter A. Shewhart</u>. The cycle can be used in various ways, such as running an experiment: PLAN (design) the experiment; DO the experiment by performing the steps; CHECK the results by testing information; and ACT on the decisions based on those results.

<u>The life Cycle of a QI Project</u>
Now that you have had a chance to evaluate your system, what is it you plan to do and how will you do it? In order to proceed, you need to have two things clearly in hand, those two things are; an objective which can be clearly articulated and the information to back it up.

<u>Overview of less common EMS CQI Models</u>

- Rapid Cycle Improvement (RCI)
- Quality Incident Stress Debrief (QISD)
- Just in Time Training (JIT)
- CE and Remediation

Rapid Cycle Improvement

<u>What is Rapid Cycle Improvement (RCI) ?</u>
Rapid cycle improvement (RCI) is traditional quality improvement (PDCA) process except the work is accelerated to be ready to implement within a 90 day cycle. When should RCI be initiated? RCI is most applicable to issues within a system which require timely resolution due to their high risk or high frequency attributes. RCI is highly suitable for EMS.

<u>Phase 1: Initiation</u> (days 1 to 5)
    The RCI Oversight Group initiates the RCI process by recognizing problem. At this point, a RCI Task Team facilitator and a team leader is designated.

<u>Phase 2: Preparation</u> (days 6 to 20)
    RCI Task Team is formed to meet and collaborate on developing an improvement statement. During this phase, the issue is broken down into steps where each step is reviewed. Quality Indicators are developed along with data and any other evidence to support the RCI project improvement statement.

<u>Phase 3: Validation</u> (days 21 to 30)
    The RCI Task Team completes this phase by clearly articulating a project improvement statement which is presented along with supporting evidence to the RCI Oversight Group. The RCI Task Team receives full approval and support from RCI Oversight Group to move forward on the RCI project.

Phase 4: Evaluation (days 31-50)
> During this phase specific action steps are developed through team consensus in response to improvement measures.

Phase 5: Authorization (days 51-60)
> These improvement measures reported by the RCI Task Team leader to the RCI Management Group for authorization to move forward to the next phase. Barriers and aids analysis is performed. Final action plan is approved.

Phase 6: Implementation (days 60-90)
> The action plan and steps are then initiated and implemented into the organization. Feedback is obtained through collection of data and evaluation of applicable quality indicators.

Phase 7: Confirmation (90 days and beyond)
> The before and after feedback is obtained and presented to the RCI Management Group for review and decision making. Based upon the judgment, discretion and authorization of the RCI Management Group, the project can be extended, terminated or recommended for a new RCI cycle.

Facilitating through Leadership

Few skills are more important and more difficult to teach than the ability to lead and facilitate consensus amongst a group of stakeholders and subject experts. These are perhaps the most important and valuable skills a Quality Manager can build and enhance.

Consensus decision making is an alternative to "top-down" decision making. Top-down decision making occurs when leaders of a group make decisions in a way does not include the participation of all interested stakeholders. Quality principles demand that their leaders obtain input and have an open the deliberation process with the involvement of the all stakeholders and participants. Proposals are collaboratively developed, and full agreement is a primary objective.

Consensus decision making is a process used by groups seeking to generate widespread levels of participation and agreement. The process of deliberation has many common elements that are definitive of consensus decision making. These include:

- Include as many stakeholders as possible in group discussions
- All participants are allowed a chance to contribute to the discussion
- The group develops proposals with input from the entire group
- The goal is to generate as much agreement as possible; a group using a consensus process makes a concerted attempt to reach full agreement
- Participants are encouraged to keep the good of the whole group in mind. Individual preferences should not obstructive the progress of the group

The Decision Making Process

Reaching a decision on the quality of system performance requires patience and good information that the decision makers trust. The better the information and the higher the quality of the presentation of the information, the easier it will be to reach a decision. Even a decision to not do anything is just as valuable as one where an initiative is launched. Leading a team through a formal decision-making process requires considerable skill and experience. Below is a decision-making model which is recommended as a guide for leading a quality team through a decision process. Please be reminded that it is just as important to have consensus amongst the decision-makers as it is to actually reach the decision.

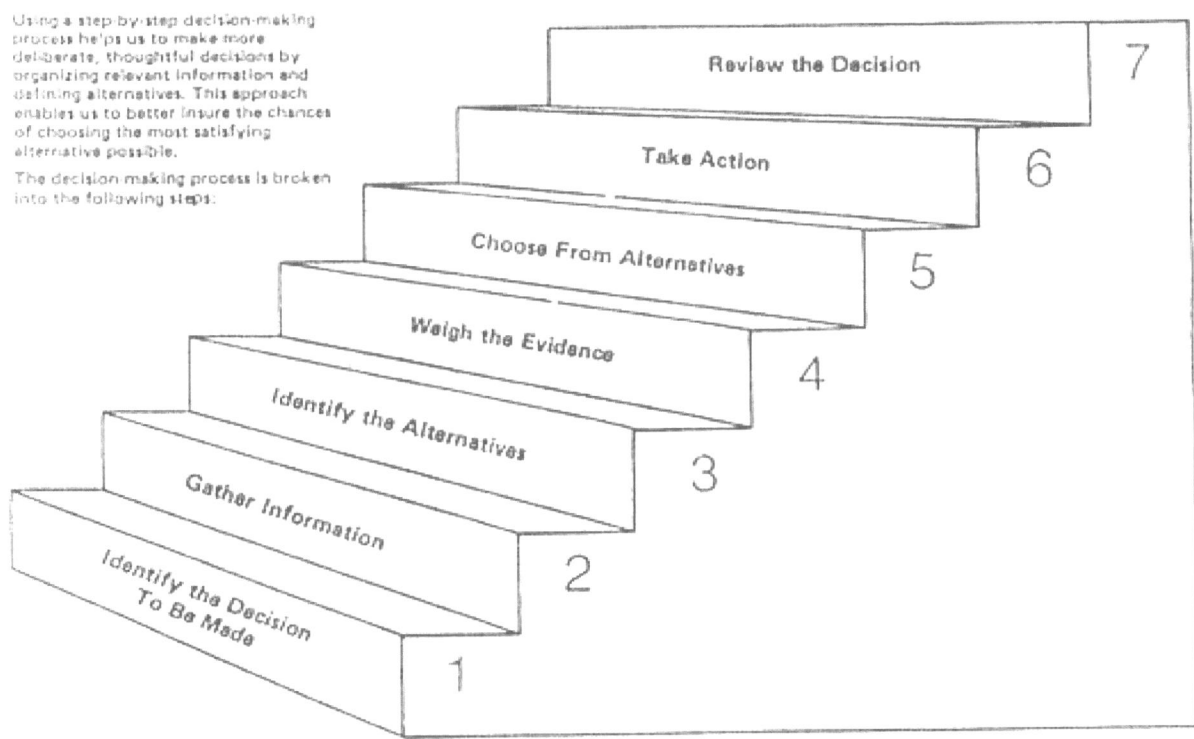

DECISION-MAKING MODEL

Using a step-by-step decision-making process helps us to make more deliberate, thoughtful decisions by organizing relevant information and defining alternatives. This approach enables us to better insure the chances of choosing the most satisfying alternative possible.

The decision making process is broken into the following steps:

Review the Decision 7

Take Action 6

Choose From Alternatives 5

Weigh the Evidence 4

Identify the Alternatives 3

Gather Information 2

Identify the Decision To Be Made 1

Consensus

Full consensus means that all stakeholders agree and support the decision. Whereas sometimes a large group may not have 100% agreement, but do have compromise and may even have what we call **Practical Consensus** which is where the team does not completely agree but they all agree to support the decision of plan to address the problem.

Root Cause Analysis

Root cause analysis and take action of an organization's quality problems center on work processes and not people. It is systematically performed, usually as part of an improvement initiative, with conclusions and root causes that are identified backed up by documented evidence.

Objectives of a Root Cause Analysis (RCA)
- o   Identify the factors that resulted in the location, timing, nature, and magnitude of any harmful outcomes
- o   identify what behaviors, actions, inactions, or conditions need to be changed to prevent recurrence of similar harmful outcomes

Four (4) Primary Steps to Performing a RCA
1.   Identify problem statement
2.   Dissect process through flow charting and collecting information.
3.   Establish root cause (diagram, brainstorm)
4.   Make recommendations to prevent or improve.

Cause-and-Effect Analysis

Cause-Effect Diagrams
Sometimes, a problem keeps us from completing a job as well as we would like. The problem may result from long-standing policies and procedures or because of a lack of adequate equipment or facilities. These problems can become more complicated to resolve if several people are working together to complete an assignment. A cause-and-effect diagram is used to show the causes of a problem. Since there is generally more than one cause to any problem, the diagram is used to further divide causes into groups or categories. This approach often uncovers the root causes of our problem. When the root causes are identified, we can evaluate how much each cause contributes to the problem.

Constructing a Cause-and-Effect Diagram
The following steps are used to construct a cause-and-effect diagram. These diagrams are sometimes called "fishbone diagrams", because they resemble a fish skeleton when completed.
Step 1. Develop a statement of the problem. Write it down on the right side of a piece of paper (the fish head). Draw a central arrow across the middle of the page that points to the problem.
Step 2. Brainstorm a list of probable causes of the problem. Write each of these down on another sheet of paper.
Step 3. Review the list of causes and identify the major categories. Write down the names of the categories as main branches (fish bones) off the central arrow.
Step 4. Review the causes and list each under the appropriate category. If necessary, revise or expand the list of categories.
Step 5. Write down each cause as a small branch drawn off the main category branch for the category under which it falls.

Why Use Cause-and-Effect Diagrams?

Cause-and-effect diagrams can help clearly illustrate possible relationships between causes. They can be used to uncover the root causes of problems or specific bottlenecks in a work process. By arranging possible causes into categories in a diagram, we can develop a better understanding of problems and contributing factors. To prepare a diagram, we must expand our original understanding of the problem situation. Our exploration often gives us a look at the underlying assumptions of our work. While a cause-and-effect diagram is an effective analysis tool, it only helps us identify possible causes or categories of problems. Even if everyone agrees on the list, it is important to determine what is not known about each cause and how that information can be uncovered. If necessary, we must collect additional data and analyze it to identify and confirm actual causes.

Image of Cause and Effect (Hishikawa) Diagram.

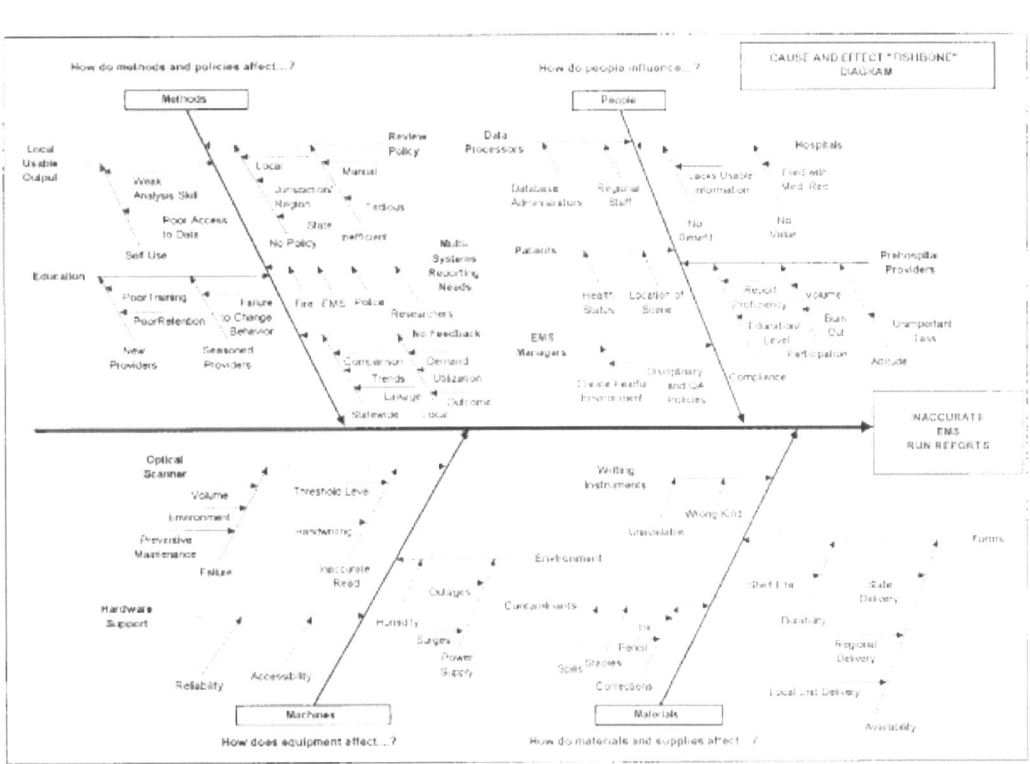

This cause-and-effect diagram was developed to identify the causes for why ambulance run reports are inaccurate. The central arrow points to the problem statement. Main branches lead to four categories of causes. These are: People, Methods, Machines and Materials. For each major causal category, there are a number of specific causes that are shown as smaller branches. When creating this diagram, a quality improvement team brainstorms a list of category specific causes and marks them on the diagram. In this figure, under the major category of methods, the QI team believes that the education programs used to teach personnel how to use the run forms properly may be ineffective in changing the behaviors of existing personnel or may not be adequate to fully inform new personnel. After listing and developing this list of "suspected" causes, the team would decide which causes are most influential and worth pursuing

Flowcharting

Every day in EMS systems, hundreds of tasks are completed in order to meet specific objectives. Much of our work flows between departments, offices and other organizations. It is easier to see how specific tasks and activities contribute to our mission if we can picture the whole process. A flowchart illustrates the activities performed and the flow of resources and information in a process.

Why Use Flowcharts?

An EMS organization pursuing quality improvement is constantly looking for ways to improve the effectiveness and efficiency of its work. "Effectiveness" means producing the required results or output when needed. "Efficiency" means simply producing those results or outcomes the first time with minimum resources. In order to generate ideas on how to be more efficient and effective, it is helpful to define and document how activities are actually performed Flowcharts are useful for this purpose.

Flowcharting

Flowcharts can be useful to identify activities in a process that reduce our effectiveness and efficiency. For example, some activities may be redundant or repeated, others may be unnecessary. Activities may be performed in sequence, when they could be conducted at the same time to reduce the overall time for the process. Flowcharts can be used to identify conditions that cause delays and bottlenecks. This can bring focus to problems at various points within the process that need further evaluation and improvement.

High Level Flowchart

A high level flowchart illustrates how major groups of related activities, often called "sub processes", interact in a process. Typically, four to seven sub processes are shown in a flowchart. By including only basic information, high level flowcharts can readily show an entire process and its key sub processes. An example of a high level flowchart is shown in Figure 1. The four sub processes are: EMS system access; information gathering and triage; pre-arrival instructions; and dispatch.

Detailed Flowchart

A detailed flowchart provides a wealth of information about activities at each step in a sub process. An example of a detailed flowchart for two of the access and dispatch sub processes is shown below. It shows the sequence of the work and includes most or all of the steps, including rework steps that may be needed to overcome problems in the process. A quality improvement team can increase the detail to show the individuals performing each activity or the time required to complete each activity. If necessary, the link between various points in the sub process and other high level flowcharts of the process can also be shown.

How to Draw a Flowchart

Flowcharts are drawn using these symbols as building blocks. A square or rectangle identifies a step (task, activity) in the process. The name of the step is written inside. Decision: A diamond identifies a decision or branch point in the process. Each path emerging from a decision block is labeled with one of the possible answers to a question that is posed at this point in the process.

An arrow indicates the sequence and direction of flow within the process. This is usually the transfer of an output of one activity to the next (where it becomes an input). Output/Input: A parallelogram identifies a material or information output or input from an activity. The name of the output (input) is written inside. A circle is used to indicate a continuation of the process flow elsewhere on the same page or on another page. The same label written on the connector symbol appears on another connector where the process flow continues.

Activity blocks are the most common elements of a flowchart. They can be arranged in serial or parallel paths depending on how activities are actually performed. Decision blocks indicate conditional situations where the output of an activity needs to meet certain criteria before the process can continue. If the criteria are not met, a different set of activities follow. This is often called "re-work" and is drawn as a feedback loop in the flowchart.

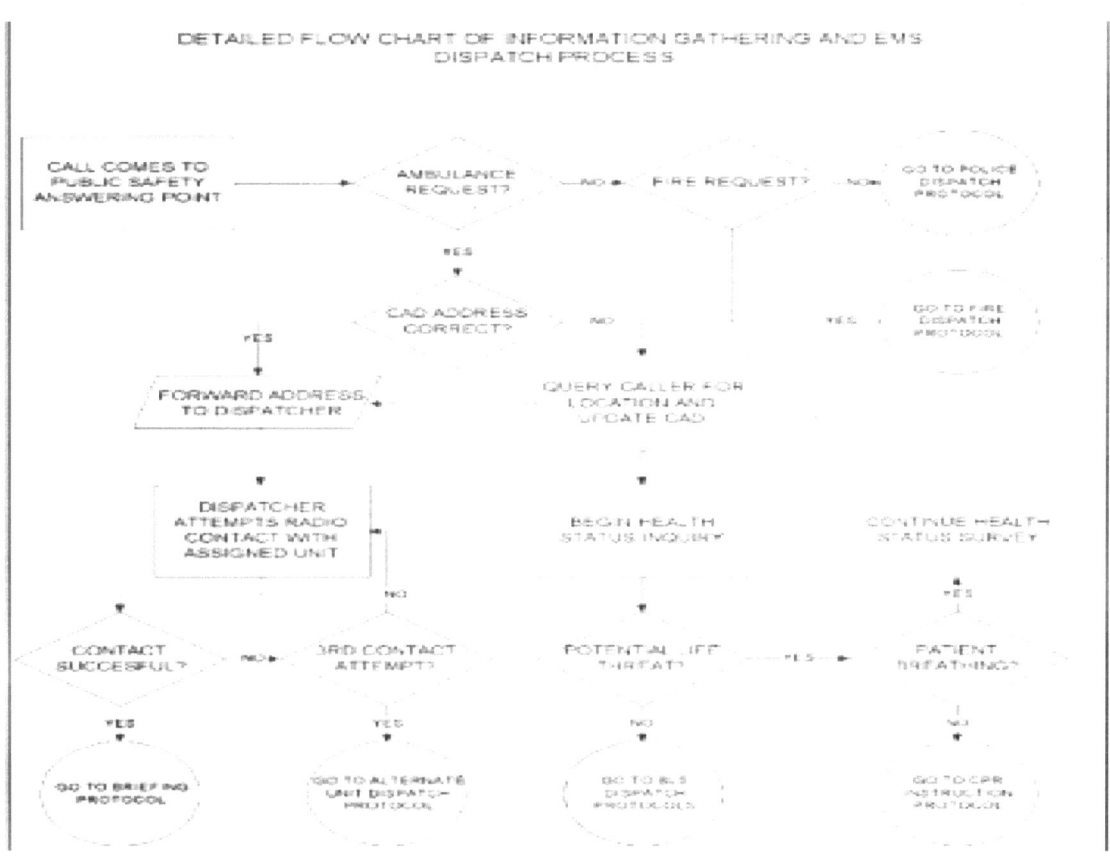

See appendix 4 for an overview of flowcharting shapes and how they are used

Fundamentals of Flowcharting Analysis

Part of the process of dissecting the root cause of a problem requires the use of flowcharting to break down steps and involve the entire team's activities. Each shape represents an activity type or process in the entire activity that is being reviewed. Below is a breakdown of each shape and corresponding activity.

The Five Whys?

The core part of the Root Cause Analysis is the part where you are you are brainstorming the problem statement and asking why up to five times. What caused the fire? Grease in a pan. Why did the grease cause the fire? Because the stove caught it on fire. Why did the stove start the fire? Because it was on too high and no one was watching it? Why was it on high with no person there? Because the lady went to answer the door with the pan on the stove while it was going at high temperature. So the final root cause could be leaving the frying chicken alone on the stove. Now we have a clear improvement that we can make.

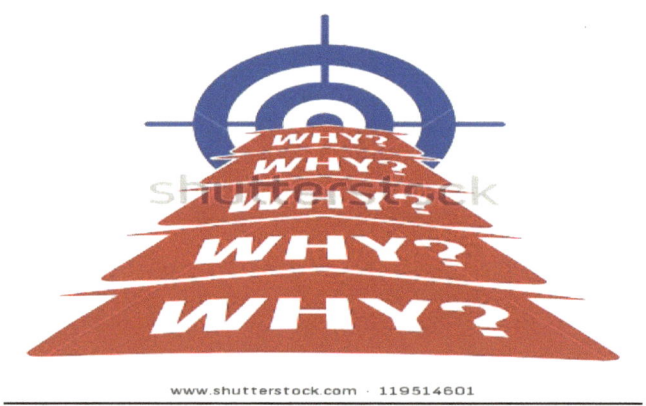

www.shutterstock.com · 119514601

Causal Factors

A causal factor is any element associated with the incident that, if corrected, could have prevented the incident from occurring or would have significantly mitigated its consequences. It could also be a barrier or safeguard that was either not in place or was in place, but was ineffective at preventing the incident.

RCA Process : Problem - Solution Matrix

During the brainstorming phase of the 5 whys, it is sometimes helpful to use a matrix to help you record and understand your answers. Below is a Root Cause Mapping Tool/Matrix

Causal Factor 1	Root Cause Mapping	Recommendations
Category: People Description- Chicken left unattended while cooking	• Cooking material unattended • Answer doorbell • Stove on	• Policy not to leave cooking material for any reason • Minimize time away unattended • Policy to turn off heat source when unattended
Category: Environment Description- Stove temperature was high with open flame	• Cooking with high temperature	• Reduce temperature from 450 to max 300 degrees

The Problem Statement

At the end of any well executed evaluation and decision making process stands a clear and specific identification of the problem or as we in the quality world like to call it; "The Challenge" before us to improve. So it is critical that once an improvement opportunity is identified, it needs to be clearly articulated in a format that all can see and all stakeholders agree upon. The specific of how it will be addressed in terms of objectives and timelines is left to those who will write the final plan or "Initiative". But again, in order for the team to plan ahead, they must first have a clearly articulated, data driven and consensus supported problem statement. Note: To see an example of a completed Problem Statement form - see Appendix 7 of this textbook.

The Quality Initiative

Initiative is all about taking charge. An *initiative* is the first in a series of actions to accomplish a specific goal. This process requires the motivation and support to get things done and take on accountability.

Once a decision is reached, it should be recorded and archived. If the decision is that the performance is safe and acceptable, it should so be noted and archived into the meeting minutes. If the decision is to take action, a task team should be appointed by documenting the appointed members and leaders (see the resource appendix at the back of this document for an example of a task team improvement sheet).

Whatever approach or improvement model (PDCA, Rapid Cycle, etc) a group chooses, the CQI Task team should have clear objectives for improvement and an improvement statement. See resource appendix for example of improvement statement which clearly identifies the goal of the task force and the objectives. The indicator should continue to be monitored and be readily available to the team at all times and through the entire improvement cycle.

Unfortunately, it has been my experience that implementation is one of the "weaker" links in the chain of processes which make up a quality initiative. For the most part, we are pretty good at obtaining information and determining what isn't working well or as well as we would like it to work. We are even pretty good about deciding what to do about it. But just like those of us who own lawns know, just because the length of the grass indicates we need to do something and we have a plan and the tools to do it, it isn't always easy to sustain the expectation of a well-manicured lawn. It takes energy and commitment (not to mention money) to make it happen. The following are some important points to assess when moving forward on an initiative; is there a grass roots commitment? Do you have the full backing of upper management and administration behind your project? This may be the time to stop and check on these two important steps in the implementation process. One of the ways to do this is to develop a specific action plan that defines the objectives of the project clearly and sets a specific but realistic timeline. These items should be presented to administrative oversight and to the working team once more for support and approval.

Planning and Implementing

There is no short term schemes to make quality and continuous improvement happen. Continuous improvement initiatives are always a work in progress and always in transition going form good to better. Planning and sustaining an initiative is the pivotal point in a quality improvement project. Just as in decision-making, after the decision is made by the stakeholders, consensus needs to be sought after and attained for all parts of the planning or action plan to address the challenge to improve.

Pioneers in quality improvement have shown that it takes between five and 10 years to achieve breakthroughs in quality and to build continuous improvement into an organization's culture. Planning and implementation strategies must be built to be long term and enduring.

Organizations that embrace quality improvement look at processes across the entire organization and do not compartmentalize issues into silos. Implementing a culture of continuous quality improvement means that changes can take place anywhere and at any level within the organization.

So planning should include the development of an initiative with a long term commitment not only by the people performing the activity but by the people who support the process from the top-down and from the bottom up.

Note: An Action Planning form that supports the planning process of this stage in the project development is available in appendix eight (8) of this textbook.

Quality Incident Stress Debrief (QISD)
This is a formal "defusing" and peer driven analysis of a difficult or complicated call. The concept borrows from the more well-known ideas of Critical Incident Stress Debriefing (CISD) in that it is done in real time and as soon as possible after the incident occurs. It is field based and utilizes peer driven techniques to dissect the incident and select areas or recommendations for improvement. There is no psychological defusing involved, it is entirely looked at as a chance to review, dissect without fault and making changes to improve the incidents in the future. This program works particularly well with Multi-Casualty events or other unusual or high stress EMS events. The process includes a follow up performed by the facilitator to provide learning points and any initiatives to improve going forward.

Just in Time Training (JIT)
This type of improvement process fits well with RCI and other initiatives where there is some urgency and simplicity to implementing the change or improvement as soon as possible. Examples of this type of implementation technique would include what is commonly called "tailgate training" where the people being trained are at the actual worksite just before they begin their shifts or tasks.

Continuing Education (CE) and Remediation.
CE as part of a Performance Improvement Plan (PIP) is currently the   most common and possibly the least effective form of improvement initiative. It is weak because it tends to be used on individuals whom are seldom truly the root cause of the problem. It is also the easiest to implement. A paramedic makes a dosage error on a cardiac case is often told to go take a class in ACLS, etc, when the problem was really that the packaging of the drug calls for several thinking step's that don't work well in the heat of the battle. Instead of taking the time and effort to look at the system and make it less burdensome on the paramedic, it is easier and we don't have to do as much if we just say "go take a class". Don't get me wrong, there are indeed times when CE and remediation are good directions to go, but as far as being effective in getting change or improving a process in the system, it is weak.

Sustaining the Gain

Again, it is important to mention the importance of a tenacious follow up and sustainment plan. In many cases, I have seen this phase fall off on the gains simply because no one was paying attention. They were assuming the problem or improvement issue was simply over and done. This is why I consider the sustaining phase of a quality improvement program as possibly the "weakest" link in the entire process. The use of quality indicators is a vital component for keeping up with the difficult job of sustaining a successful quality initiative campaign. Simply because a project was successful and has been implemented, does not mean that it has been fully integrated into the culture and work force.

Continuous checking is important. Establishing "red flags" to tip quality personnel of relapses and signs that old habits are hard to fully break become as important as the original evaluation phase. In some ways, the sustaining phase of a quality project becomes even more valuable because all the effort and expense has taken place and we now simply just need to hold the line on the gain. The development or modification of quality indicators becomes important and should be developed in the same way, but now with timelines and milestones built into the measuring of long term improvement. Perhaps the indicator may now need to be classified and archived as a core or tertiary indicator based upon the consensus of the quality leadership team.

Perhaps just as important is the organization's need to share the experience with others who are in the same or similar circumstances. The results of the project and the corresponding indicators should be shared with all who are stakeholders as well as those customers that may not be directly tied to your organization. One suggested way to accomplish this task is through transparency and the development of an Initiative Status Board which can be posted in plain view directly in the workplace.

The table below is an example of a tool often used to help monitor and sustain CQI initiatives. It is called an initiatives status board and contains examples of initiatives currently in different phases of implementation or monitoring. The board is posted in conspicuous places and used to make the project transparent, specific and real to stakeholders and their customers. The board clearly shows the project action plans, steps in the process, deadlines, expected outcomes and accountability. It also serves as a historical document of the overall story of the Initiative.

2013-14 Quality Initiatives
"Our Quality Stories in Detail"

PROJECT TITLE	OUTCOME STATEMENT	Phase I Staff Research & Review	Phase II Task Team QLC Review	Phase III Approval & Planning	Phase IV Implement	Phase V Monitoring	Phase VI Sustainability
Pre-Hospital "Push-Out" program	To increase the efficiency and verify implementation of system changes or improvement projects which are pushed out through our training	Staff is currently gathering data to see how well recent projects such a Ped med Safety and new Treatment Guidelines were pushed.	Action Plan -to be presented for approval at June 2013 meeting				
Pediatric Medication Safety	To reduce pediatric medication errors less than 1%	-Data received & reviewed by EMS Staff --Published in EMS Best Practices	Completed QLC review June 14, 2011. -Task team assigned and action planned approved	-New weight based measuring prototype and ped tx cards approved 7-2011, costs determined and ordered	Meeting 12/27, training session for distribution 12/28, All equipment and training distributed by	Staff to visit random stations to assure field personnel understand project objectives. Maintenance	Data to be collected and measured in the same way over the next six months will be evaluated at 6 month intervals.
Inter-Facility Transfers of Critical Trauma Patients	To significantly reduce the inter facility transfer times of critical trauma patients in CCC	- Data collected - Task Team to be appointed	Task team of local ED physicians and Trauma Center staff have had Adhoc meetings to develop	Team approved new transfer center at JMMC. Transfer center went into operation	Adhoc meeting to be scheduled in 2013 to check status		

The Third Component of
An EMS Quality Program

EMS Safety Events
Reporting

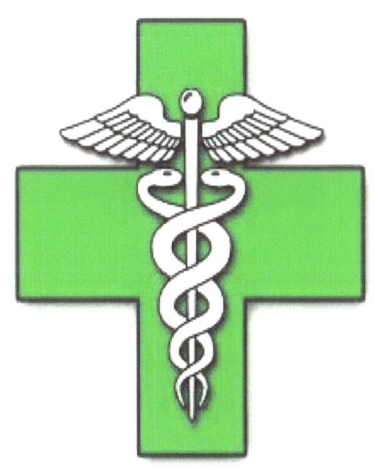

Defining Patient Safety and EMS Events Reporting

<u>What is a Patient Safety Event?</u>
While the healthcare industry has been developing and improving the concepts of patient safety for several years now, it is only recently that the prehospital healthcare discipline (EMS) has begun to emphasize the reporting, analysis, and prevention of medical errors that may lead to adverse healthcare events.

EMS has been pretty efficient at taking on the old-school role of the "enforcer". For the past decades, EMS has been doing the old quality assurance model. Looking for things that went wrong and blaming people for it. In my opinion, quality assurance was misnamed; it should have been called "penalty assurance".

Over the past decade, the health care industry has learned the hard way that the mistakes that threaten our patients are far more likely to be the natural consequence of poorly designed systems and accordingly rarely (less than 10%) the fault of an incompetent person.

Therefore, our primary focus should be on the system that supports the EMS provider and not on the individual that executes it. Specifically, our efforts should be on designing systems that can intercept errors before they cause harm to the patient. Again, more that 80% of medical errors are caused by bad systems, not bad people. Simply put, it's all about how to design processes that make it easy for people to do things right, and hard to do things wrong.

*Source: *WHO Patient Safety Curriculum Guide for Medical Schools*. Geneva, Switzerland: World Health Organization; 2008:99. The following chart shows the scale and effects of patient safety issues worldwide

Data on adverse events in health care from several countries

	Study	Study focus (date of admissions)	Number of hospital admission	Number of adverse	Adverse event rate (%)
1	United States (Harvard Medical Practice Study)	Acute care hospitals (1984)	30 195	1 133	3.8
2	United States (Utah–Colorado study)	Acute care hospitals (1992)	14 565	475	3.2
3	United States (Utah–Colorado study)[a]	Acute care hospitals (1992)	14 565	787	5.4
4	Australia (Quality in Australian Health Care Study)	Acute care hospitals (1992)	14 179	2 353	16.6
5	Australia (Quality in Australian Health Care Study)[b]	Acute care hospitals (1992)	14 179	1 499	10.6
6	United Kingdom	Acute care hospitals (1999–2000)	1 014	119	11.7
7	Denmark	Acute care hospitals (1998)	1 097	176	9.0

In reviewing the previous table, it is obvious that not all errors reach patients or cause harm. However, we must still learn and take on these events as opportunities to improve. Furthermore, though an error may be discovered and corrected, many times it may eventually slips through again because of other problems in the system that were not considered or explored.

Moreover, errors that lead to serious patient harm are rarely the result of just one error involving one person. Again, I point out that there are typically a series of errors or breakdowns in process, most of which have probably been occurring for some time, just not all at once. Unfortunately, in some instances there is no clear source of error to be found and still that does not diminish the harm to the patient. All errors or untoward events must be kept on the front burner with "hawk-like" monitoring by the patient safety organization.

Bearing all these points collectively, we must use a systems approach to analysis and improvement and avoid blame and punishment. A systems approach involves recognizing that the design of systems and processes are the major contributors to EMS Events and errors, not the individuals working within those systems. To improve, there must be examination of these systems—processes, procedures, equipment, organizational culture—that can lead to error. We must never consider patient harm as unavoidable or we will not learn how to improve.

So how does this strategy of conducting patient safety and EMS Events reporting differ from the concepts of system evaluation and improvement presented in the prior two sections of this book?

In a general sense, there isn't a great difference. We still approach the issue or event as a systems problem first, and we are focusing our energy on improving the process and not providing an individualistic approach to preventing these events from occurring again. Our primary focus is on protecting the patient from any potential or further harm. This approach relies on an open and self- reporting system that points out or catches events that may be of harm to patients. The reports are compiled, processed and evaluated for trends and clusters in the system. The review and action portion of the process is limited to whether or not it is a significant event and then whether or not it is system wide. Once these determinations are made, then the process follows traditional PDCA models discussed in the prior two sections.

The hallmark guiding principles of an EMS patient Safety and EMS Events Reporting program include at a minimum the following;
- Establish patient safety as a visible commitment to the "putting patients first" philosophy
- Move from blaming people to improving processes
- Improve use of technology to prevent and detect errors or events
- Use data to identify and measure improvements

Above all else, commitment to the care and improvement of EMS Patient service should be shared as much as possible with other healthcare providers. The common saying amongst many quality circles is; "Steal shamelessly and share generously." Passing on important and relevant patient safety information to our fellow providers can help to improve and possibly eliminate many patient safety concerns.

Confidentiality & Protections
EMS confidentiality protections when performing patient safety has been a weak link and a point of contention in some cases. In most cases, patient safety and review of actual incidents is considered part of a comprehensive "Quality Review Process" with formal ties to similar activities done within hospitals or trauma committees where sections of the penal codes and other statutory laws protect the exposure of the committee activities from disclosure to civil litigation. The contemporary position by most EMS organizations is proceeding as though the same protections offered to the healthcare industry in general are inclusive to prehospital care as well. There still remains much more to be tested and understood regarding the application of confidentiality and discovery statutes in this area of quality improvement.

Organizational Committee Structure of a Patient Safety Review Committee

Just like the system evaluation and quality improvement process must have a working structure and processes in place and because the patient safety process should be separate from CQI program, we recommend a separate internal structure with key stakeholders as the primary facilitators and members of a regular committee or group. The following is an example of the org structure and workflow for an organized patient safety program. In this example the safety committee is called the Internal Review Committee.

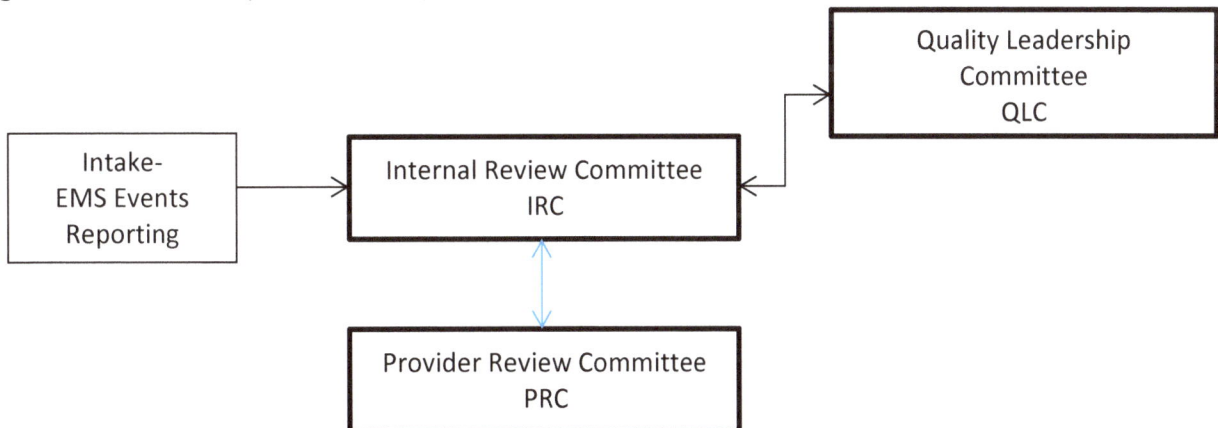

Internal Review Committee (IRC)
This is led by EMS System staff which includes the CQI staff who intake all reports and do the initial review. This group is advisory to the Medical director.

Provider Review Committee (PRC) once a report has been reviewed it goes to the provider agency for their respective review and action as necessary. CQI Staff from the IRC meet with individual providers PRC at regular intervals to clear and clarify events. When the event or issue has been resolved, the outcome is fed back to the IRC where it is closed; the type and details of the case are entered into a data base for tracking and trending by CQI staff. Reports on the activities, trends and issues for the IRC are shared with the system wide QLC..

EMS Safety Events Reporting & Workflow

Processing of EMS Events Reports

All staff and provider staff involved in the patient safety program are trained on the following steps used to process an EMS Events.

1.	Intake:	Events are reported on a standardized form (see appendix) and can be submitted via internet, phone, fax or U.S. Mail.
2.	Triage:	Report is initially reviewed by CQI staff to determine if immediate threat to public or licensing action immediately required -If so action taken immediately.
3.	Assign:	A reviewer is appointed as a single point of contact.
4.	Review:	The report is reviewed by staff using a standardized form to review
5.	Consult:	The report may then be given to provider agency to complete a more thorough review and make recommendations for action.
6.	PRC:	The final summary from the review and recommendations may then be exchanged and negotiated at the Provider Review w committee (PRC) as needed.
7.	IRC:	The report is discussed and recommendations approved.
8.	Med Dir.	Final summary of review and recommendations from the review staff are presented to the Medical Director for approvals or modifications.
9.	Closure:	The event then receives final approval for action and recommendations
10.	Record:	Once closed the event report is archived into data base.
11.	Trending:	The data base is sampled and reviewed for trends and clusters as identified.
12.	Report:	The information on frequency and types as well as trending is reported to QLC system wide every six months.

High Risk Events Reporting

Patient Safety should include the reporting of high risk events that "could" happen but haven't yet. In other words, while many EMS events tend to be reported after the fact, it is just as important to encourage our system participants to report situations which appear to be "just waiting to happen". High risk or hear miss events that indicate a chance of happening. The idea being that prevention of a serious patient safety event is a much more powerful tool than the fixing of an event after it has occurred. Because of this basic common sense principle, Quality Managers are encouraged to be progressive and develop pre-emptive safety initiatives and promote the reporting of high risk events before they occur as a part of the comprehensive EMS events reporting system.

Confidentiality & Protections

Many states around the nation do not provide adequate confidentiality, or peer review protections for EMS agencies and providers. Each program should consider all available protections and barriers to performing this portion of quality improvement. One possible solution to overcome protection barriers may be to contract with an established Patient Safety Organization (PSO). These PSO's offer federal-based confidentiality protection resources for your safety and quality improvement work.

The Just Cause Culture

Each organization should have policies and guidelines which lead the activities of the IRC and PRC as the review process is carried out. The technique for reviewing each events reporting may slightly differ depending on the nature and severity of the event. One of the guiding principles in reviewing and resolving EMS patient safety events is the concept of "Just cause". While this process has become most used by employers over the last decade, it has similar application to the EMS review process when trying to obtain the pertinent information and action on a situation while balancing the rights of an individual involved in a review. The following is a brief description of the just cause approach to reviewing EMS events with serious issues. Especially, if this event has led to the one in ten chance that the error was caused by an individual.

Once an event is clearly recognized as a potential licensing or certification revocation, the reviewer should immediately recognize that while the event is still reviewable under the CQi-patient safety process, the authority to investigate and take action now rests with the statutory agency and the report should now go to them for follow and closure. The patient safety process can continue to review confidentially and once the statutory action has been completed, can reach an analysis and take action in the system to prevent the event from repeating. The Just-cause processes are generally applicable to employee-employer relations, but can be recognized as a reasonable approach to assuring the rights of an individual who is up for review.

The process can be reduced to seven categories which are as follows;:
1. Adequate warning
2. Reasonableness
3. Completeness of investigation
4. Objectivity of investigation
5. Proof of infraction
6. Uniformity of Application of Rules
7. Reasonableness of discipline.

When any one of these requirements is not met, the discipline should be dismissed. Unlike the Legal System, however, precedent has only persuasive authority in the labor dispute context. Each contract and working environment is viewed to stand alone in the disciplinary arena. The following is a closer look at each category;

1. Adequate Warning

   Did provider know the rule existed? For example, the provider may have transported a patient to a hospital that is further and lower level of specialty than the one the patients ended up at. The provider is reprimanded and suspended for not following the new policy to transport to closest and highest level of care. Was the policy clearly posted and distributed? If it was in a Policy and Procedures Manual, did the provider sign anything saying he read and understood the Policy? If the answer to these questions is "No," how would the provider know about the Policy? Even if the policy was posted or a provider signed a document, the provider still has the right to adequate warning of the action he may face, including loss of license or employment

2.   Reasonableness
     Reasonableness is defined as "Fair, proper, or moderate under the circumstances. Reasoning comes down to attitude. I recommend arguing for unreasonableness only in concert with other tests for just cause, or as a last resort.

3.   Completeness of Investigation
     How do you know that the provider committed the infraction? Was an informant involved? Was he observed by a third party? We have had much discipline tossed because management didn't have their ducks in a row at hearing. For example, if a product was damaged and records indicate that the accused was the last to handle the product, is that adequate to show guilt? We have shown many times that it isn't. In the damaged product example, we look at when the employee was last in the area, when the damage was discovered, and who else had access to the area. We look at surrounding circumstances to establish reasonable doubt. Generally, if the employer cannot produce a "smoking gun," the employee should be ok.

4.   Objectivity of investigation
     Did we look at this situation more closely than when the same or similar infractions occurred? Producing evidence that the infraction was treated lightly in the past places the burden on us to show why the employee is being closely observed now. Unlike classic discrimination claims, where singling out must be shown in the context of membership in a protected class, Just Cause defense only requires showing that the employee was unduly scrutinized. The second prong of the Fair Investigation Doctrine is whether other employees were investigated, and whether other explanations were considered. The crux of the Doctrine is to assure that the employee isn't being targeted.

5.   Proof of Infraction
     Related to Completeness of Investigation, proof of Infraction is a cornerstone of Due Process. Defining proof, however, isn't necessarily held to the strict Rule of Law. As in Reasonableness of Rule, the "proof" rests in what the arbitrator accepts as fact.

6.   Uniformity of the Rule's Application
     As with Objectivity of Investigation, Uniformity of Application exists to assure that the suspect isn't singled out. If you can show that others did the same thing, management knew or should have known about it, and discipline was nonexistent or less severe, then you can show a violation of the Just Cause Test. Just Cause is the single most powerful employee protection.

7.   Reasonableness of Discipline
     Again, as with reasonableness in general, the discipline issued by the authority must match the level of severity and be the same in nature and intensity as other similar events. So essentially, the discipline should be consistent and fit the infraction.

Glossary of Quality Terms & Nomenclature

Action Plan – A written plan with objectives and steps to bring action with an organization to change or initiate an improvement in a process or outcome indicator.

Bar Chart - A graphic presentation which represents quantities through the use of bars of uniform width but heights proportional to number being represented.

Benchmarks: Known and accepted results. Quality measures of performance (structures, process, outcomes) often used synonymously with indicators, measures and metrics

Benchmarking - using known results of similar data measurements or tests as an impetus for achieving or surpassing a desired goal for improvement.

Best Practices - using the best known results of similar data

Beta Testing - To perform an exercise in obtaining and analyzing a specific indicator.

Bi-variable – indicator end result is in a reporting value that requires two sources of data.

Causation - the results of tests which are applied to a set of data points plotted on a process control chart. The tests determine whether or not a "special cause" exists within the data set and can explain unusual

CEMSIS - California Emergency Medical Services Information System.

Classification – Catalog titles given to indicators.

Continuous variable - indicator end result is in a reporting value that has infinite potential such as a measurement of time or length. Often measured by a benchmark potential such as the 90th percentile.

Control chart - Graphic presentation of a line graph specifically used to track the trend or performance of a process over time. Useful in demonstration process variability.

Core Indicator - The lead indicator being analyzed. Core indicators are composed of several sub-indicators (smaller indicators), which are major contributing factors to the final core indicator result.

Core Indicator Index # - Index number as classified by state EMS vision project.

Core Indicator name - Name given to the core indicator.

(D) Symbol - Represents denominator.

Data Aggregation - To blend all data together.

Data Blinded - Withholding identification of data sources or subjects.

Data Sampling - Obtaining information from a data source.

Data Linkage - Relating to two separate data sources or data banks to the same subject.

Data Stratification - Breaking down of the whole into smaller related sub-groups.

Denominator (D) Inclusion Criteria - Specific data element/points needed to perform the data query as related to the specific indicator.

Denominator (D) Data Source - The instrument used to capture the data.

Description of Indicator Formula – description of how indicator results are mathematically derived and determined.

Display Format - The medium or style in which the final indicator results are displayed

Domain of Performance - The category of performance being evaluated.

EMS Service Provider - An organization employing EMT-I, EMT-II, or EMT-P certified or licensed personnel for the delivery of emergency medical care to the sick and injured at the scene of an emergency and/or transport to a general acute care hospital.

EMS System Quality Improvement (EMS-QI) - An organized and formal effort to continually achieve superior outcomes through ongoing evaluation of performance indicators by system users and providers within an organized EMS Health Delivery System.

Effectiveness - How well a system is meeting an expressed objective or benchmark.

EQIP- EMS Quality Improvement Plan. A plan put together by an EMS service provider which details all aspects of their quality improvement activities.

Frequency – How often a system is meeting an expressed objective or benchmark.

Frequency of Display – How often a specific indicator unit should be displayed.

Histogram – A visual representation of the spread or distribution of the data categories. Data are represented by bars of equal width or category and the height of these bars indicate the relative number of data points in each category.

Just In Time Training (JIT): A training style which emphasizes providing the training to the employee as they enter the working environment. Usually short and concise and done where the employee or worker would most likely be when the subject task would be done.

Indicator Specification Sheet (ISS) – A sheet of paper or electronic form which contains the standardized and accepted definitions and parameters for a quality indicator.

Indicator Formula Numeric Expression – Mathematical expression of how indicator result are determined and derived.

Indicator Reporting Value – The numeric value of the indicator result.

Lean – an established quality improvement program pioneered by the Toyota Corporation which focuses on work flows and cutting out waist.

Line graph – A visual display of data for comparison. Specific data points are entered by numbers are connected by a line. Useful in demonstrating a data pattern.

Linkage Options – The different elements that may be used to link two separate data sources or banks.

Metrics: Quality measures of performance (structures, process, and outcome). Term often used synonymously with indicators, measures and benchmarks.

Measures: Quality measures of performance (structures, process, and outcome) Term often used synonymously with indicators, measures and benchmarks.

Measures of central tendency – Values that describe the middle or majority of the data.

Measures of dispersion – Values that describe how the data is spread out from the average.

Mean – (Average) Sum of all data divided by the number of data points.

Median – The middle of all ranked and counted data points.

Minimum Data Values – The smallest number of data values which must be available to perform a measure and analysis.

Mode – The value repeated most often in the raw data.

(N) Symbol – Represents the numerator.

NEMSIS – National Emergency Medical Services Information System

Numerator (N) Data Source – The instrument used to capture the data.

Numerator (N) Inclusion Criteria – Specific data element/points needed to perform the data query as related to the specific indicator.

Objective – A description of the information that indicator is seeking to measure.

Outcome – The result of activities (processes) performed by attributes (structures) within a system; measures of intended system performance.

Pareto chart – A way of organizing data to show what major factors make up the indicator being analyzed. Useful in showing the many parts of a whole such as all the sub-indicators of a core indicator.

PDCA – Acronym for Plan-Do-Check-Act which are the four primary steps in traditional continuous quality improvement plans.

Performance Indicator – A comparison used to answer the question "how are we doing?"

Performance Measurement – The process of measuring accomplishments, as well as measuring in process parameters.

Periodic – Sampling specific data at random periods with random amounts.

Pie chart – A graphic presentation that compares relative magnitude of frequencies or parts of a whole. Useful in presenting outcome and process information.

Problem Statement: - A written description of an issue or problem which has been detected and analyzed through the use of an indicator and is ready to be evaluated by a CQI group.

Population Exclusion Criteria - Specific data element/points which may be used to exclude related data from a specified data query.

Population Denominator (D) - The overall subject that the indicator measures.

Population Subset Numerator (N) - The subset measurement of the denominator population.

Process - The repeatable sequence of actions used throughout interrelated components of a Prehospital EMS system to produce something of value.

Process variation - Evaluations to determine if variations within a process are statistically out of control.

Published References - using published results of similar data measurements or tests as beginning or starting point for achieving or surpassing a desired goal for improvement.

Range - Maximum single data value minus the minimum single data value.

Rapid Cycle Improvement (RCI) – A form of traditional (PDCA) continuous quality improvement which emphasizes a more rapid response and change cycle.

Rate - Sampling specific data at a specific time for a specific amount.

References - Information related to the indicator which may contain helpful comparisons on indicator performance, best practices or benchmarks.

Scatter diagram - A visual display showing the relationship between two variables. Useful in showing the relationship of a process to an outcome (e.g., time & survival).

Sentinel - Sampling all specific data at all times.

Single variable - indicator end result is in a reporting value that requires only one source of data.

Six Sigma – A continuous quality improvement program which focuses primarily on evaluating data and the levels of dispersion from the bell curve means.

Source - Origin of indicator development.

Special cause - The result of a statistical trending measurement which shows a cause in variation is statistically significant and warrants further evaluation.

Standard deviation - A measurement that shows how widely spread (dispersed) any set of data is from the average.

Stratification Options - Common data elements used to stratify a specific indicator.

Structure - The interrelated components forming a Prehospital system.

Success Rate - How often a specific activity (process) is performed successfully.

Sub Indicator - Smaller indicators that are contributing factors to a core indicator.

Sub Indicator index # - Index number as classified by state EMS vision project.

Sub Indicator name - Name given to subject sub-indicator.

Trending Analysis - A series of statistical tests to determine significant variation in a process

Type of Measure - Identifies weather an indicator is structural, process, or outcome.

Variation - Evaluations to determine if a process is statistically out of control.

SUGGESTED READINGS AND REFERENCES

1. Berwick DM: Continuous Improvement, N Engl J Medicine 320:53-56, 1989
2. Balestracci D; Data *Sanity: A Quantum Leap to Unprecedented Results, 3rd Edition.* Englewood, CO. Medical Group Management Association (MGMA), January 2009.
3. Cummings RO. The Utstein Style for uniform reporting of data for out of hospital cardiac arrest. Annals of Emerg Med. Jan 1993. 22: 37-40
4. Deming. WE: Out of Crisis. Cambridge, MASS: MIT Press International: 1982
5. Donabedian A. Definition of quality and approaches to its assessment. Ann Arbor, MI Health Administration Press; 1980
6. Donabedian A. The quality of Healthcare. JAMA. 1988: 260. 1743-1748
7. Drummond MF, Obrien BJ, Stoddard GL, Torrance GW. Methods for the economic evaluation of health programs. NY. Oxford University Press: 2003
8. Eastman JN. Walz BJ, Fear in the Workplace. Journal of EMS(JEMS) 1993: 18 (5) 53-67
9. Evans A. Avoiding Ten Benchmarking Mistakes. www.benchmarkingphs.com.ac
10. EMS Insider La Sage Taigman; March 2015; Vol 42, #3
11. EMSA; Emergency Medical Services System Core Quality Measures, EMSA, State of California; #166 – Appendix E, April 2013.
12. EMSA; Emergency Medical Services System Quality Improve Prog Model Guidelines, EMSA, State of California; #164, March 2004.
13. Gausche M, Lewis RJ, Stratton SJ et al. Effect on out of hospital pediatric intubation on survival and neurological outcome:. JAMA 2000; 283: 112-16
14. Gunderson, M; Performance Indicators, In Lerner EB, Pirrallo R, Swor R; Evaluating and Improving Quality in EMS. NAEMSP. 2009: 99-113
15. Haynes, J: Quality Improvement in EMS: EMS WOLD EXPO; Oct 2012.
16. Institute for Healthcare Improvement' Patient Safety Development Program (IHI); Conference Handbook; Orlando, FL 2011; www. IHI.org
16. Joint Commission on Accreditation of Healthcare Organizations (JCAHO) Development and Applications of Indicators in Emergency care. 2001. 52
17. Joiner B L. *Fourth Generation Management: The New Business Consciousness.* New York, NY: McGraw-Hill, 1994 [ISBN 0-07-032715-7].
18. Mazen J. El Sayed* Measuring Quality in Emergency Medical Services: A Review of Clinical Performance Indicators; Emerg Med Int. 2012: 61630. Published online 2011 October 15. : 10.1155/2012/161630 PMCID: PMC3196253
19. Mainz J. Developing evidenced based clinical quality indicators. International Journal of Quality in Healthcare. 2003: Suppl 1: i5-i11
20. Mears G, Zalkin J, In: Kuehl A. EMS information systems and the future of EMS data base. Prehospital Emergency Care. 2001; 6: 123-130
21. Moore L. Performance Measurement in EMS. In Lerner EB, Pirrallo R, Swor R; Evaluating and Improving Quality in EMS. NAEMSP. 2009: 80-98
22. North Carolina Prehospital Medical Information Systems. www.premis.net
23. National Highway Safety Administration (NHTSA). EMS Agenda for the Future: 1996. www.nhtsa.dot.gov/people/injury/ems/agenda. Dec 4 2007.
24. National EMS Information System. www.nemsis.org
25 NHTSA Version 3.0 Uniform Data Set. 2014. www.nemsis,org

SUGGESTED READINGS AND REFERENCES

26.. Sobo E, Andriese S, Stroup C, Morgan D, Kurtin P, Developing Indicators for emergency medical services (EMS) system evaluation and quality improvement; a statewide demonstration and planning project. Joint Commission; (JCAHO); Journal of Quality Improvement, 2001: 27: 138-154.

27. Stroup, Craig: Developing and Utilizing Quality Indicators for Emergency Medical Services Evaluation and Improvement. CEMSPI; Center for EMS Performance Improvement. October 2014.

28. NHTSA. Leadership Guide to Quality Improvement in EMS

29. Stickle. R: Developing a Quality Improvement Program in EMS. Advanced Leadership Issues in EMS. Pages 9 http://www.usfa.fema.gov/pdf/efop/efo33925.pdf; National Fire Academy

Organizations & Resources

The following were used to help develop this textbook and are excellent resource material for further reading, contact or reference.

1. California LEMSA CQI Coordinators Committee
2. Institute for Healthcare Improvement (IHI)
3. UC Davis Extension Health Care Analytics Program
4. EMS Healthcare Analytics (UC Davis Healthcare)
5. National Association of EMS Quality Coordinators (NAEMSQC)

Resource Appendices

1-6

Job Title: Quality Manager

Job Description: The Quality Manager is the primary leadership role in any organized quality program. This position is responsible for the overall coordination and activities related to all there components of the system; evaluation, improvement and safety. This position requires a strong formal education and training in the three areas of quality. Experience within the respective CQI program system is very valuable. The manager should have strong analytical, communication and team building skills. Leadership through consensus building also be a priority skill. This position is often filled by a Physician, Registered Nurse or Paramedic. The Quality Manager may also be the Medical Director if qualified.

Qualifications: Bachelor's Degree from accredited four year University. Current license as a EMT-Paramedic or Registered Nurse. Minimum of six years FTE as a practitioner on a 911 emergency response unit or in an urban hospital emergency department or intensive care unit. Certification or course completion in quality training from nationally recognized CQI training program such as Institute of Healthcare Improvement (IHI) or equivalent.

Abilities and Skills: Ability to perform technical and professional writing on a word processor, manage and manipulate data on a basic excel platform. Develop and present charts and graphical information via Microsoft power point. Strong leadership, facilitating and consensus building skills required.

Job Title: Medical Director

Job Description: The CQI medical Director position is a leadership position
                             where the director works in collaboration with the Quality
                             Manager and team to provide oversight and medical
                             direction to the comprehensive program. The Medical
                             Director obtains and evaluates quality information and
                             provides direction and interpretation as to the level of
                             quality in the system and helps decide whether action to
                             improve and sustain is required. The Medical Director helps
                             facilitate and reach consensus amongst community CQI
                             leadership.

Qualifications: Current license as Physician with a minimum of six years FTE
                             as a practitioner in an urban hospital emergency
                             department or intensive care unit. Certification or course
                             completion in quality training from nationally recognized
                             CQI training program such as Institute of Healthcare
                             Improvement (IHI) or equivalent desired.

Abilities and Skills: Ability to perform technical and professional writing on a
                             word processor, manage and interpret data on a basic
                             excel platform. Strong leadership, facilitating and
                             consensus building skills required.

Job Title: Data System Manager

Job Description: This role is primarily to work with the Quality manger and
                           CQI groups to help develop and implement important CQI
                           level measures. This position is a person who has been
                           trained and has demonstrated competency in the overall
                           data systems management and who shall be responsible
                           to implement, maintain, troubleshoot, operate, query and
                           provide data mining in order to produce reports which
                           support the day to day CQI program operations. The Data
                           System Manager shall report to the Quality Manager.

Qualifications: minimum six years FTE and evidence of formal training as a
                           data system manger. Experience in providing excel data
                           system based reports and charts.

Abilities and Skills: Strong written and oral communications experience
                           desired. Ability to provide technical assistance and speak
                           to large audiences a plus.

.

Appendix 1
CQI Job Descriptions

Job Title: Field Training Officer

Job Description: Each program should have Field Training Officers (FTO) who
                          are official leaders in the quality improvement program
                          and who work in collaboration with the EMS agency to
                          provide input and assist in the implementation of quality
                          initiatives in the system.

Qualifications: Minimum of six years FTE as a field paramedic on a 911
                          emergency response. Certification or minimum of 8 hr.
                          training or course completion in quality training from
                          nationally recognized CQI training program such as
                          Institute of Healthcare Improvement IHI) or EMS equivalent.
                          The FTO shall be appointed by the provider service and be
                          approved by the CQI program Quality Manger.

Abilities and Skills: Strong written and oral communications experience
                          desired. Ability to provide technical assistance and speak
                          to large audiences a plus. Ability to interpret and
                          understand complex graphs and charts. Instructional
                          experience desired.

Guide to Determining Which Chart to Use

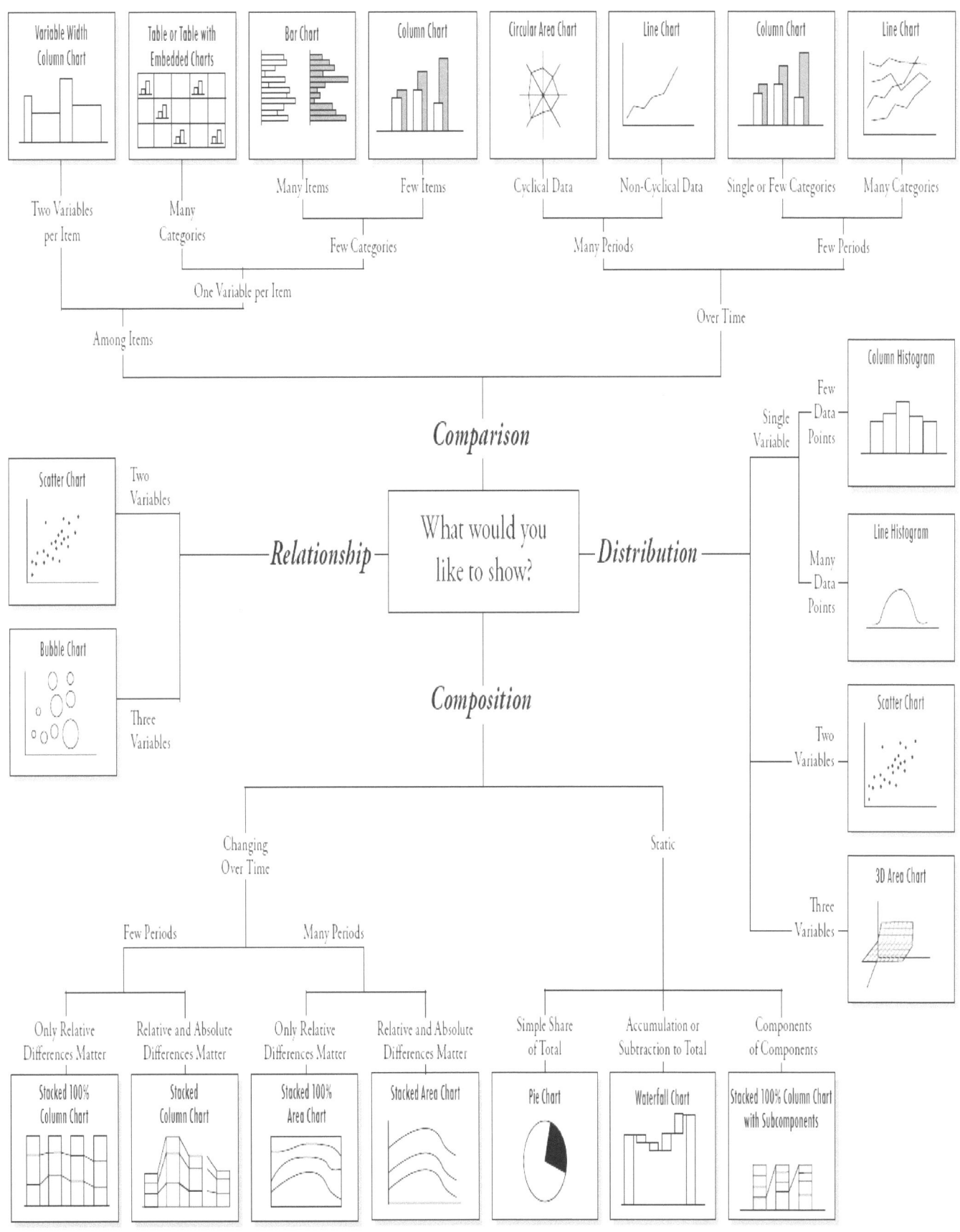

Flowcharting Symbols

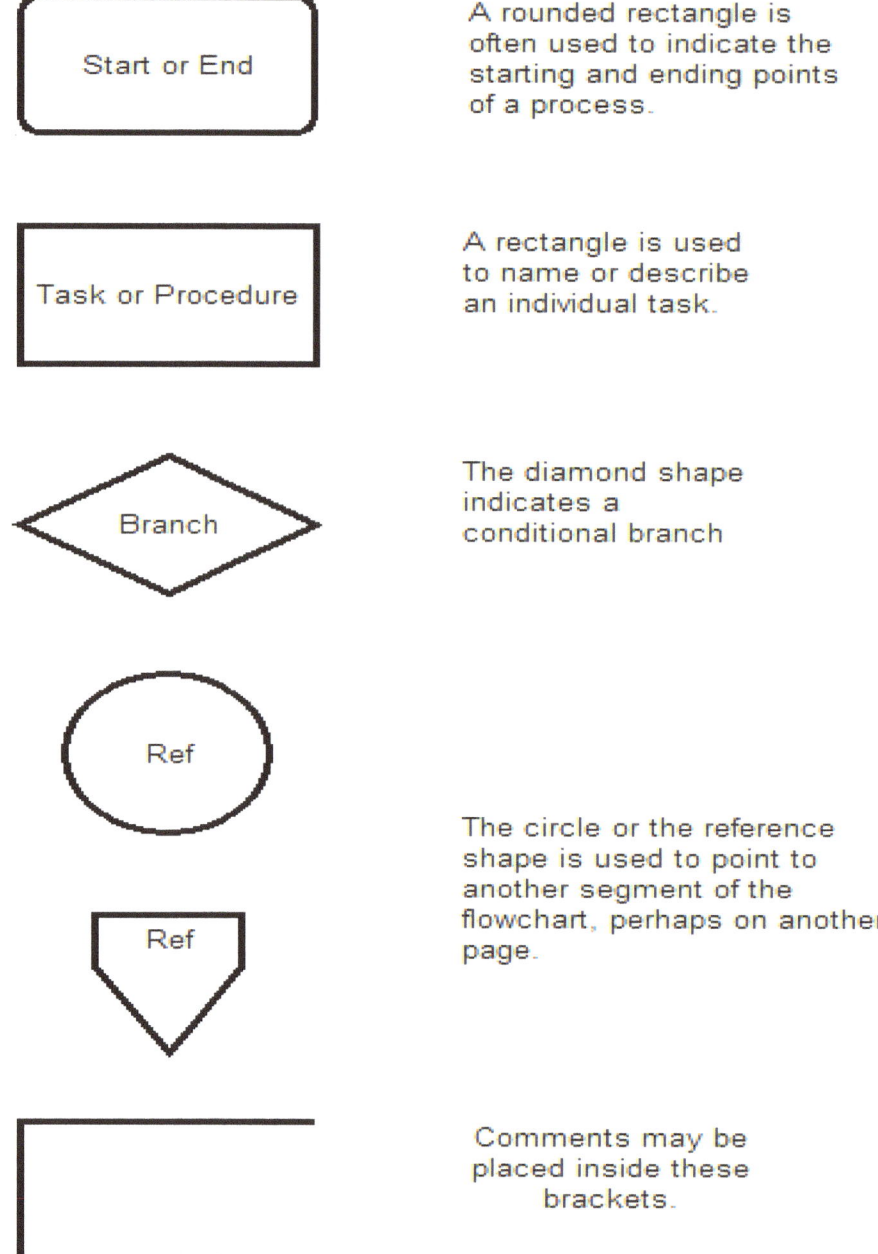

Commonly Used Flowchart Shapes

Start or End — A rounded rectangle is often used to indicate the starting and ending points of a process.

Task or Procedure — A rectangle is used to name or describe an individual task.

Branch — The diamond shape indicates a conditional branch

Ref / **Ref** — The circle or the reference shape is used to point to another segment of the flowchart, perhaps on another page.

Comments may be placed inside these brackets.

<u>Rules of Conduct</u>

- Try to attend all meetings
- Respect other peoples time
- Be prepared and organized
- Take turns speaking and listening
- Postpone side conversations
- Silence your devices
- Keep an open mind
- Participate constructively
- Blame the process, not the person
- Do what you say you'll do

CQI INDICATOR EVALUATION FORM

INDICATOR #   _____

INDICATOR TITLE: _____

	YES	NO
Does the indicator show special cause or potentially unsafe results	____	____
Is there an opportunity to increase patient safety?	____	____
Is the indicator below performance expectations?	____	____
Is there an opportunity to increase performance levels?	____	____
Is there an opportunity to institute a cost saving initiative?	____	____
Is there an opportunity to institute a operational efficiency initiative?	____	____
Does the indicator need further review or stratification?	____	____
Should an Action Plan Initiated?	____	____

Please explain any "YES" answer below;

_____

_____

_____

_____

_____

_____

LEAD REVIEWER NAME   _____   DATE: _____

COMMITTEE GROUP NAME: _____

ATTACH ACTION PLAN AS INDICATED

Electronic Version Available at: _____

EMS Indicator Update Project

CEMSIS Data Table Request Form

The purpose of this form is to assist with the process of generating CEMSIS reports for EMS quality indicators. CAEMSQI project data will be provided in the form of a data table, and more than one table may be required to address a single indicator. To request a data table, a minimum of five form sections must be addressed:

Request Form Sections
1. Basic report information
2. Table population
3. Measures
4. Perspective and audience
5. Dimensions

1- Basic Report Information

#EMS163 Indicator Number _____

Indicator Name _____

Report Number (tbd) _____

Report Title _____

CAEMSQI group contact: _____

2- Table population

Using CEMSIS elements and field values, define the base population (i.e. denominator) for this data table. List specific exclusion criteria as needed.

3- Measures

Describe the base measure for this data table. Include a formula if applicable. Also, use CEMSIS elements and field values to define the numerator population as needed.

4- Perspective and audience

Report level (grain)		Audience	This report will be used by	
	State	Identifiable data	EMSA	Hospital
	Local EMS Agency	De-identified data	EMSAAC	
	Hospital	Public data	Local EMS Agency	
	Provider		Provider	

EMS Systems Data Request Form
last update April30, 2012

Problem/Issue Statement

RCI Project #   #_____

RCI Project Name: Pediatric Med Errors

Problem –Improvement Statement:

"Reduce the number of annual field pediatric medication errors to none (0) for a minimum of eighteen (18) consecutive months."

Objectives:

❑ To implement new tool (color coded "Broselow type" tape and county approved matching pedi medication "quick reference cards) to determine and confirm the 5 rights of the pediatric patients.

❑ To make pedi-med reference tool available on both adult paramedic jump bags and in the shelves of the response units.

❑ Provide and communicate a clear mechanism for personnel to replace their field handbook when lost or damaged.

❑ Verbalize to confirm the dose and "how you got there" as a step in the administration of medications to all pedi-patients.

❑ Follow implementation of above changes with in-house training component.

❑ Explore how to integrate smart phone protocol application into work environment.

Team Leader Name: _____
Team Facilitator Name: _____
Date: _____

Action Plan Form

RCI

Action/Implementation Plan

RCI Project # _____

RCI Project Name: _____

Implementation Statement and deadlines:

_____
_____
_____
_____

Action Steps: **Who? & by When?**

❑

❑

❑

❑

❑

❑

❑

❑

❑

❑

❑

❑

Team Leader Name: _____

Team Facilitator Name: _____

Date: _____

Patient Safety EMS Events Reporting

Policies & Procedures

I.   PURPOSE

Patient Safety Events (PSE) are regularly reported and acted upon by the Emergency Medical Services Agency. The purpose of this policy is to provide and identify the process that shall be used to address all PSE. This procedure shall be conducted as a component of the Quality Improvement Process and shall be considered a confidential and protected process of our comprehensive CQI program.

II. **POLICY AND PROCEDURE**

The following process shall be used to assure that all Patient Safety Events (PSE) are addressed and acted upon by the EMS agency as part of a comprehensive quality improvement and feedback loop for our customers and constituents.

1.   Patient Safety Event (PSE) occurs

2.   PSE is recognized and acknowledged by care givers or other patient advocate

3 . PSE Form completed and sent to EMS via email, fax, mail or by telephone.

     (form filled out by staff)

4.   PSE routed initially to CQI Coordinator for review and assignment.

5.   EMS Medical Director and/or appropriate EMS Staff advised of PSE as necessary

5.   PSE assigned to appropriate EMS Staff for resolution and follow up.

6.   PSE is reviewed by assigned EMS Staff.

7.   PSE is evaluated and resolved through CQI process at regularly scheduled Provider Patient-Safety Conferences (**PPC**). (These conferences will be coordinated by EMS and involve a collaborative effort to review, resolve and provide follow up to the PSE with only the agencies involved in the event.

8.   PSE resolution or PIP shall be reported to regularly scheduled Internal Patient-Safety Committee (**IPC**) formerly the IRC, this committee shall remain open only to designated EMS staff members.

9.   PSE Resolution submitted back to CQI Coordinator for closure

10. PSE resolved and closed.

11. PSE basic information is recorded into data base.

12. PSE form and all other records related to PSE destroyed.

Appendix 3
EMS Patient Safety
EMS EVENT REPORTING FORM
PART A

Instructions: Reporting is encouraged by all who encounter an actual or potential patient event, system concern, or exemplary care delivered that may have had an impact on the quality of care or a potential safety event occurring within the County EMS system. Please provide a concise description of the event. No patient names or other personal information should be reported on this form.

Incident#: (For EMS use only)	PCR#
Date of Event:	Approximate Time:
Event Location:	Form Initiated by (Name/Title/Organization):
Receiving Facility:	Contact Info:
Others involved with the incident. Please include name and contact info:	

Details of Event: (provide facts, observations, and statements. (Use addendum if needed) ☐ Addendum Attached

Submit completed form to County QI coordinator.

Appendix 3
EMS Patient Safety
Instructions on completing EMS Events form

- This form is to be completed for every reported EMS event.
    - This information should originate from the provider involved and may be submitted anonymously
    - Assure that the notification process described in Policy # has been followed.
    - Provide a concise description of the event.
    - Individuals receiving the report should complete a brief summary of findings and disposition of the event and submit to the appropriate QI personnel.
    - Events that need follow-up should be conducted in coordination with QI personnel.
    - Oversight for the EMS event reporting process is the responsibility of each involved agency's QI staff in conjunction with the Quality Improvement Committee.
- In reviewing the event consider the following questions
    - What are the facts of the events? Be objective.
    - What factors lead up to or contributed to the event?
    - What consequences resulted from the event?
    - Could the event been prevented? How?
    - What can be learned from the event?
    - What required actions need to be taken?
- EMS Event Criteria requiring Agency notification:
    - Any EMS event that leads to or has the potential to cause a community concern.
    - Threat to public health and safety (as defined by Health and Safety Code 1798.200)
        - Any of the following actions
            - Fraud in the procurement of any certificate or license under this division
            - Gross negligence, repeated negligent acts
            - Incompetence
            - The commission of any fraudulent, dishonest or corrupt act related to the qualification, functions and duties of prehospital personnel
            - Conviction of any crime which is substantially related to qualification, functions and duties of prehospital personnel
            - Violating or attempting to violate directly or indirectly, or assisting in or abetting the violation of or conspiring to violate, any provision of this division or regulations adopted by the authority pertaining to prehospital personnel.
            - Violating or attempting to violate federal or state statute or regulation which regulates narcotics, dangerous drugs or controlled substances
            - Addiction to the excessive use of or misuse of alcohol beverages, narcotics dangerous drugs or controlled substances
            - Functioning outside the supervision of medical control in the field care system operating at the local level, except as authorized by any other license or certification
            - Demonstration of irrational behavior or occurrence of a physical disability to the extent that a reasonable and prudent person would have reasonable cause to believe that the ability to perform the duties normally expected may be impaired.
            - Unprofessional conduct exhibited by any of the following
                - Mistreatment or physical abuse of any patient resulting from force in excess of what a reasonable and prudent person trained and acting in a similar capacity while engaged in the performance of their duties.
                - Failure to maintain confidentiality of patient medical information except as permitted by law Section 56-56.6 of the Civil Code
                - Commission of any sexually related offense under section 290 of the penal code.

Appendix 3
EMS Patient Safety
EMS EVENT REPORTING FORM
PART B
TO BE COMPLETED BY REVIEWING AGENCY

1. Could this event cause a community concern or a threat to public health and safety? ☐ No ☐ Yes

    If yes, notify Medical Director and as soon as possible.

2. Could this event be possible cause for certificate or license action? ☐ No ☐ Yes

    If yes, notify licensing division and Director as soon as possible.

    Immediate efforts to resolve this issue:

    _____

    _____

☐ N/A

Incident Type

☐ Operations

       ☐ Contract ☐ Dispatch ☐ MCI ☐ System ☐ Police ☐ Intra-agency ops ☐ Other

☐ Clinical

       ☐ Medical ☐ Behavioral ☐ STEMI ☐ Stroke ☐ Trauma ☐ Peds ☐ Skills ☐ Other

---

EVENT REVIEW ASSIGNED TO:

_____PHC

RESULTS OF REVIEW: (attach addendum to back if needed) ☐ Addendum Attached

RECOMMENDATIONS: (Use addendum to back if needed) ☐ Addendum Attached

REVIEWED BY IRC?   ☐ No ☐ Yes
REVIEWED BY MED DIR? ☐ No ☐ Yes
RESOLVED?   ☐ No ☐ Yes
CLOSE DATE: _____

EMS Continuous Quality Improvement Plan Template

Notice: The following is intended to be a general guide and templet for EMS organizations to develop an internal written continuous quality improvement (CQI) plan. It is not intended to represent the requirements or the regulations nor has it been endorsed or sponsored by any private, public, or other governmental regulatory agency. Organizations which are developing their plans are advised to check with their local EMS authorities or established quality groups in their local jurisdictions for their specific requirements prior to developing their CQI plans. This template was written to be comprehensive. Organizations using this template should consider it a guide to pick and choose what is appropriate for their organization and customer requirements.

Emergency Medical Services Quality Improvement Plan

Template

Submitted by

(Insert Your Provider or Agency Name)

Date of Submission

(Add provider or company name)

Date Submitted: _____

PART I   Introduction

Introduction: Mission, Vision, Scope of Service
(**Provide a** program **description** including the **service providers** mission and vision, the types of services provided, size, etc,)

_____

_____

_____

_____

PART II   Basic CQI Principles

The following Quality Improvement Plan serves as **primary structure and guidelines of this** (add provider or company name) to continuously improve the quality of the treatment and services **we** provide.

- Quality improvement is a systematic approach to continually evaluating and improving services and assuring patient safety as a priority at all times. (*Provider or Organizations Name*) implements this approach to quality improvement is based on the following principles:
- *Customer Focus:* High quality organizations focus on their internal and external customers and on meeting or exceeding needs and expectations.
- Patient Outcome: Services are committed to reducing the pain, suffering, morbidity and mortality of all sick and injured patients in the prehospital and emergency transport setting.
- Empowerment: Our programs involve people at all levels of the organization for improving quality and puts forward the basic CQI concept that most problems are caused by the system and not the process.
- Leadership: Strong leadership, direction and support of quality improvement activities by the governing body and CEO are key to performance improvement. This involvement of organizational leadership assures that quality improvement initiatives are consistent with provider mission and/or strategic plan.

PART II   Basic CQI Principles - cont

- Information Driven: We believe successful QI processes create feedback loops, using data to inform practice and measure results. Fact-based decisions are likely to be correct decisions.
- Statistical and Process Control Tools: For comprehensive CQI, tools and methods are needed that foster knowledge and understanding. Our CQI organization will use a defined set of analytic tools such as run charts, cause and effect diagrams, flowcharts, Pareto charts, histograms, and control charts to turn data into information.
- Prevention and Sustainability: CQI seeks to design good processes to achieve excellent outcomes rather than fix processes after the fact.
- Continuous Improvement: We strive to continually review and improvement of our processes. Small incremental changes do make an impact, and we can almost always find an opportunity to make things
- That the treatment provided incorporates evidence based, effective practices; The treatment and services are appropriate to each patients-customer's needs, and promptly available when needed;
- Risk to patients-customers and others is minimized, and errors in the delivery of services are prevented;
- Patients-customers receive individual needs and expectations are respected; consumers – or those whom they designate – have the opportunity to participate in decisions regarding their treatment; and services are provided with sensitivity and caring;
- Procedures, treatments and services are provided in a timely and efficient manner, with appropriate coordination and continuity across all phases of care and all providers of care. (Add or subtract principles as your organization appropriate)

PART. III.   Continuous Quality Improvement Activities.

Quality improvement activities emerge from a systematic and organized framework for improvement. This framework, adopted by the leadership, is understood, accepted and utilized throughout the organization, as a result of continuous education and involvement of staff at all levels in performance improvement. Quality Improvement involves three primary activities: System Evaluation, Quality Improvement Initiatives and rigorous Patient Safety reporting and monitoring.

1. **System Evaluation:** Measuring and assessing the performance information through the collection of data and analysis of that data by the conversion of that data to standardized quality measures/indicators developed with end user and subject expert consensus.
2. **Quality Improvement Initiatives:** Making decisions based upon analysis of measures/indicators and conducting quality improvement initiatives **which may include** taking action where indicated, including the design of new services, and/or improvement of existing services.
3. **Patient Safety:** Providing an open process for reporting, acting and monitoring patient safety issues. The tools used to conduct these activities are described in Appendix A, at the end of this Plan.

PART IV   Leadership and Organization

Leadership.
The key to the success of the Continuous Quality Improvement process is leadership. The following describes how the leaders of the (add provider or company name) clinic provide support to quality improvement activities.

The Quality Improvement Committee
provides ongoing operational leadership of continuous quality improvement activities at the clinic. It meets at least monthly or not less than ten (10) times per year and consists of the following individuals: (List titles of committee members. The membership should include a patient/consumer advocate for both adult and pediatric level patients and at least one family member for a past patient as well as one member from the public at large.

(Indicate the Chairperson, members and characteristics of each member of the Committee.)

_____

_____

_____

_____

The responsibilities of the Committee include:

- Developing and approving the Quality Improvement Plan.
- As part of the Plan, establishing measurable objectives based upon priorities identified through the use of established criteria such as those determined by conducting a valid customer requirements study for improving the quality and safety of services.
- Developing quality measures/indicators of quality on a priority basis.
- Periodically reviewing and accessing information based on the indicators, taking action as evidenced through quality improvement initiatives to solve problems and pursue opportunities to improve quality.
- Establishing and supporting specific quality improvement initiatives
- Reporting to the public or other oversight agencies or boards.
- Formally adopt specific plans and approaches to Continuous Quality Improvement *(such as Plan-Do-Check-Act: PDCA).*
- Supporting and guiding implementation of quality improvement activities at the clinic.
- Reviewing, evaluating and approving the Quality Improvement Plan annually.

(Describe how leadership will support clinic's QI Program.)

_____

_____

_____

_____

The Leaders support QI activities through the planned coordination and communication of the results of measurement activities related to QI initiatives and overall efforts to continually improve the quality of care provided. This sharing of QI data and information is an important leadership function. Leaders, through a planned and shared communication approach, ensure the **community, customers,** staff, recipients and family members have knowledge of and input into ongoing QI initiatives as a means of continually improving performance.

This planned communication may take place through the following methods;

- Story boards and/or posters displayed in common areas
- Recipients participating in QI Committee reporting back to recipient groups
- Sharing of the clinic's annual QI Plan evaluation
- Newsletters and or handouts

Please describe your clinics method and/or mechanism for communication to recipients, staff and leadership.

_____

_____

_____

_____

PART V   Goals and Objectives

The Quality Improvement Committee identifies and defines goals and specific objectives to be accomplished each year. These goals include training of clinical and administrative staff regarding both continuous quality improvement principles and specific quality improvement initiative(s). Progress in meeting these goals and objectives is an important part of the annual evaluation of quality improvement activities.

The following are the ongoing long term goals for the (add provider or company name) QI Program and the specific objectives for accomplishing these goals for the year _____ . (Indicate the current year.)

- To implement quality measures/indicators to assess key processes or outcomes;
- To bring managers and staff together to review measures/indicators and major clinical adverse occurrences to identify problems;
- To carefully prioritize identified problems and set goals for their resolution;
- To achieve measurable improvement in the highest priority areas;
- To meet internal and external customer requirements;
- To provide education and training to managers and staff;
- To develop or adopt necessary tools, such as practice guidelines, consumer surveys and quality indicators.

List here your goals and objectives for the current year.

PART VI.   Performance Measurement

Performance Measurement is the process of regularly assessing the results produced by the program. It involves identifying processes, systems and outcomes that are integral to the performance of the service delivery system, selecting indicators of these processes, systems and outcomes, and analyzing information related to these indicators on a regular basis. Continuous Quality Improvement involves taking action as needed based on the results of the data analysis and the opportunities for performance they identify.

The *purpose* of measurement and assessment is to:

- Assess the stability of processes or outcomes to determine whether there is an undesirable degree of variation or a failure to perform at an expected level.
- Identify problems and opportunities to improve the performance of processes.
- Assess the outcome of the care provided.
- Assess whether a new or improved process meets performance expectations.

Measurement and assessment *involves*:

- Selection of a structure, process or outcome to be measured, on a priority basis.
- Identification and/or development of performance indicators for the selected structure, process or outcome to be measured.
- Aggregating data so that it is summarized and quantified to measure a process or outcome.
- Using process analysis as one of the techniques to look at stability and level of performance
- Assessment of performance with regard to these indicators at planned and regular intervals.
- Taking action to address performance discrepancies when indicators indicate that a process is not stable, is not performing at an expected level or represents an opportunity for quality improvement.
- Reporting within the organization on findings, conclusions and actions taken as a result of performance assessment.

Selection of a Performance Indicator.

A *performance indicator* is a quantitative tool developed through consensus of users and providers that provides information about the performance of a structure, process, or outcomes. Selection of a Performance Indicator may be based on the following considerations:

- Relevance to mission - whether the indicator addresses the population served
- Clinical importance - whether it addresses a clinically important process that is:
  - high volume
  - problem prone or
  - high risk

Characteristics of a Performance Indicator.
Factors to consider in determining which indicator to use include;

- Data Driven: the relationship between the indicator and the structure, process, or outcome being measured
- Validity: whether the indicator assesses what it purports to assess
- Resource Availability: the relationship of the results of the indicator to the cost involved and the staffing resources that are available
- Customer Oriented: the extent to which the indicator takes into account individual or group feedback and preferences
- Meaningfulness: whether the results of the indicator can be easily understood, the indicator measures a variable over which the program has some control, and the variable is likely to be changed by reasonable quality improvement efforts.
- For purposes of this plan, an indicator(s) comprises core elements and is defined using an indicator specification sheet (ISS) such as the one attached in this appendix of this plan.

  The following represents each performance indicator currently in use by the provider, along with the corresponding descriptors.

_____

_____

_____

_____.

<u>Assessment.</u>
Assessment is accomplished by comparing actual performance on an indicator with:

- Self over time.
- Pre-established standards, goals or expected levels of performance.
- Information concerning evidence based practices.
- Other clinics or similar service providers.

(List here the assessment strategies you will use. See APPENDIX for examples of performance improvement tools.)

Section 5 – Quality Improvement Initiative
Once the performance of a selected process has been measured, assessed and analyzed, the information gathered by the above performance indicator(s) is used to identify a continuous quality improvement initiative to be undertaken. The decision to undertake the initiative is based upon clinic priorities. The purpose of an initiative is to improve the performance of existing services or to design new ones. The model utilized at (**Add provider or company name)** is called Plan-Do-Check-Act (PDCA). *(Modify the following as appropriate for your program. If you choose a model other than PDCA, describe the model here*

- Plan - The first step involves identifying preliminary opportunities for improvement. At this point the focus is to analyze data to identify concerns and to determine anticipated outcomes. Ideas for improving processes are identified. This step requires the most time and effort.
- Do - This step involves using the proposed solution, and if it proves successful, as determined through measuring and assessing, implementing the solution usually on a trial basis as a new part of the process.
- Check - At this stage, data is again collected to compare the results of the new process with those of the previous one.
- Act - This stage involves making the changes a routine part of the targeted activity. It also means "Acting" to involve others (other staff, program components or consumers) - those who will be affected by the changes, those whose cooperation is needed to implement the changes on a larger scale, and those who may benefit from what has been learned. Finally, it means documenting and reporting findings and follow up.

Section 6 – Evaluation

An evaluation is completed at the end of each calendar year. The annual evaluation is conducted by the and kept on file in the clinic, along with the Quality Improvement Plan. These documents will be reviewed by the Office of Mental Health as part of the clinic certification process. The evaluation summarizes the goals and objectives of the clinic's Quality Improvement Plan, the quality improvement activities conducted during the past year, including the targeted process, systems and outcomes, the performance indicators utilized, the findings of the measurement, data aggregation, assessment and analysis processes, and the quality improvement initiatives taken in response to the findings.

- Summarize the progress towards meeting the Annual Goals/Objectives.
- For each of the goals, include a brief summary of progress including progress in relation to training goal(s).
- Provide a brief summary of the findings for each of the indicators you used during the year. These summaries should include both the outcomes of the measurement process and the conclusions and actions taken in response to these outcomes. Summarize your progress in relation to your Quality Initiative(s). For each initiative, provide a brief description of what activities took place including the results on your indicator. What are the next steps? How will you "hold the gains." Describe any implications of the quality improvement process for actions to be taken regarding outcomes, systems or outcomes at your program in the coming year.)
- Recommendations: Based upon the evaluation, state the actions you see as necessary to improve the effectiveness of the QI Plan.

PART VII.   Quality Improvement Tools

Following are some of the tools available to assist in the Quality Improvement process.

a. Flow Charting: Use of a diagram in which graphic symbols depict the nature and flow of the steps in a process. This tool is particularly useful in the early stages of a project to help the team understand how the process currently works. The "as-is" flow chart may be compared to how the process is intended to work. At the end of the project, the team may want to then re-plot the modified process to show how the redefined process should occur. The benefits of a flow chart are that it:

1. Is a pictorial representation that promotes understanding of the process
2. Is a potential training tool for employees
3. Clearly shows problem areas and processes for improvement.

   Flow charting allows the team to identify the actual flow-of-event sequence in a process.

b. Pareto Chart: The "Pareto Principle" says 20% of the source causes 80% of the problem. Pareto charts allow the team to graphically focus on the areas and issues where the greatest opportunities to improve performance exist.
c. Run Chart: Most basic tool to show how a process performs over time. Data points are plotted in temporal order on a line graph. Run charts are most effectively used to assess and achieve process stability by graphically depicting signals of variation. A run chart can help to determine whether or not a process is stable, consistent and predictable. Simple statistics such as median and range may also be displayed.
    The run chart is most helpful in:
    1. Understanding variation in process performance
    2. Monitoring process performance over time to detect signals of change
    3. Depicting how a process performed over time, including variation.
d. Control Chart: A control chart is a statistical tool used to distinguish between variation in a process resulting from common causes and variation resulting from special causes. It is noted that there is variation in every process, some the result of causes not normally present in the process (special cause variation). Common cause variation is variation that results simply from the numerous, ever-present differences in the process. Control charts can help to maintain stability in a process by depicting when a process may be affected by special causes. The consistency of a process is usually characterized by showing if data fall within control limits based on plus or minus specific standard deviations from the center line. Control charts are used to:
    1. Monitor process variation over time
    2. Help to differentiate between special and common cause variation
    3. Assess the effectiveness of change on a process
    4. Illustrate how a process performed during a specific period.

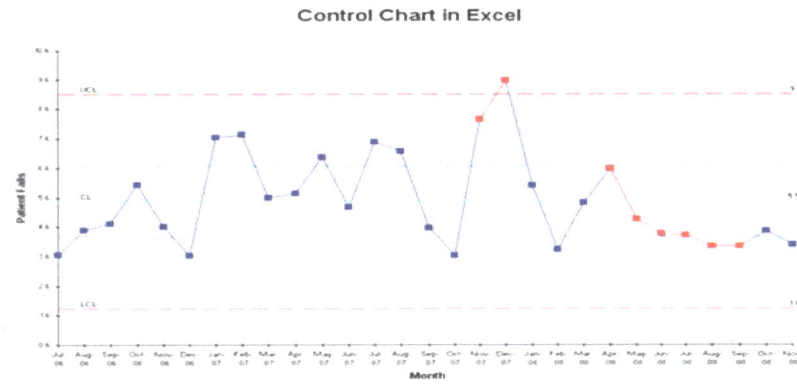

Control Chart in Excel

Using upper control limits (UCLs) and lower control limits (LCLs) that are statistically computed, the team can identify statistically significant changes in performance. This information can be used to identify opportunities to improve performance or measure the effectiveness of a change in a process, procedure, or system.

e. Bench Marking: A benchmark is a point of reference by which something can be measured, compared, or judged. It can be an industry standard against which a program indicator is monitored and found to be above, below or comparable to the benchmark.

k. Root Cause Analysis: A root cause analysis is a systematic process for identifying the most basic problems in Objectives of a Root Cause Analysis. It includes the following key components;

1. Identify the factors that resulted in the location, timing, nature, and magnitude of any harmful outcomes.
2. Identify what behaviors, actions, inactions, or conditions need to be changed to prevent recurrence of similar harmful outcomes

PART VI.   Annual Updates

The Annual Update is a written account of the progress of an organization's activities as stated in the EMS QI Program. In compiling the Annual Update, refer to the previous year's update and work plan. Describe how, how often, and who (job title) in your organization evaluates the QI Plan (annually at minimum). Annual review/updates shall include the indicators monitored, key findings/priority issues identified, improvement action plan/plans for further action, and state whether goals were met. If goals were not met, what follow-up is needed, if any?

The following reference which may be helpful in developing and organizing this plan is;

www.emsa.ca.gov/pubs/pdf/emsa166.pdf
California State EMS System Quality Improvement Program Model Guidelines, Publication Document#166; Section II Data Collection and Reporting for guidance on how to select these indicators. Refer to Appendix E: Indicator Categories, for indicators relative to your role in the EMS system. Refer to Appendix M: Quality Improvement Sample Indicators, for assistance identifying the indicators that relate to your organization.

SINGLE VARIABLE INDICATOR SPECIFICATION SHEET	
Measure Set	
Set Measure ID #	
Performance Measure Name	
Description	
Type of Measure	
Reporting Value	
Denominator Statement (population)	
Example of Final Reporting Value	
Suggested Display Format & Frequency	
Suggested Statistical Measures	☐ Mean ☐ Median ☐ Variance ☐ Mode ☐ Standard Deviation
Trending Analysis	☐ Yes ☐ No
Benchmark Analysis	☐ Yes ☐ No
References	

SINGLE VARIABLE
INDICATOR SPECIFICATION SHEET

Measure Set	Manpower
Set Measure ID #	Per # 02
Performance Measure Name	Number of Licensed Paramedics
Description	What is the number of currently licensed paramedics who work in the EMS System?
Type of Measure	Structure
Reporting Value	Numeric
Denominator Statement (population)	Current number of licensed paramedics
Example of Final Reporting Value	102
Suggested Display Format & Frequency	Table or Column Graph
Suggested Statistical Measures	☐ Mean ☐ Median ☐ Variance ☐ Mode ☐ Standard Deviation
Trending Analysis	☐ Yes ☐ No
Benchmark Analysis	☐ Yes ☐ No
References	1. County EMS Personnel Records

BI-VARIABLE INDICATOR SPECIFICATION SHEET			
Measure Set			
Set Measure ID #			
Performance Measure Name			
Description			
Type of Measure			
Reporting Value			
Denominator Statement (population)			
Numerator Statement (sub-population)			
Indicator Formula Numeric Expression			
Example of Final Reporting Value			
Suggested Display Format & Frequency			
Suggested Statistical Measures	☐ Mean ☐ Mode	☐ Median ☐ Standard Deviation	☐ Variance
Trending Analysis	☐ Yes ☐ No		
Benchmark Analysis	☐ Yes ☐ No		
References			

BI-VARIABLE INDICATOR SPECIFICATION SHEET	
Measure Set	Cardiac Arrest
Set Measure ID #	CAR-4
Performance Measure Name	% Out-of-Hospital Cardiac Arrests Survival to Hospital Discharge
Description	What is the percent (%) of those patients who experience cardiac arrest of cardiac origin after the arrival of EMS providers that survive to be discharged from the hospital over a specific period of time?
Type of Measure	Outcome
Reporting Value	% Percentage
Denominator Statement (population)	Total number of patients experiencing cardiac arrest of cardiac origin after the arrival of EMS providers over a specified period of time
Numerator Statement (sub-population)	Total number of patients experiencing cardiac arrest of cardiac origin after the arrival of EMS providers that survive to discharge from the hospital over a specified period
Indicator Formula Numeric Expression	The formula is to divide (/) the numerator (N) by the denominator (D) and then multiply (x) by 100 to obtain the (%) value the indicator is to report. Therefore the indicator expressed numerically is N/D =%
Example of Final Reporting Value	36%
Suggested Display Format & Frequency	Bar Chart; Run Chart
Suggested Statistical Measures	☐ Mean ☑ Median ☐ Variance ☐ Mode ☐ Standard Deviation
Trending Analysis	☑ Yes ☐ No
Benchmark Analysis	☑ Yes ☐ No
References	1. Utstein 2. AHA

Blank Template
Indicator Spec Sheet
Continuous Variable

CONTINUOUS INDICATOR SPECIFICATION SHEET	
Measure Set	
Set Measure ID #	
Performance Measure Name	
Description	
Type of Measure	
Reporting Value	
Continuous Variable Statement (Denominator Population))	
Example of Final Reporting Value	
Numerator Statement (sub-population)	
Indicator Formula Numeric Expression	
Suggested Display Format & Frequency	
Suggested Statistical Measures	☐ Mean ☐ Median ☐ Variance ☐ Mode ☐ Standard Deviation
Trending Analysis	☐ Yes ☐ No
Benchmark Analysis	☐ Yes ☐ No
References	

Completed Example
Indiicator Spec Sheet
Continuous Variable

CONTINUOUS INDICATOR SPECIFICATION SHEET	
Measure Set	Response & Transport
Set Measure ID #	RT# 105
Performance Measure Name	90% Scene Time Interval – Major Trauma Victim
Description	What is the time interval in minutes for 90% of the calls where a paramedic ambulance that is on scene of a patient who is a major trauma victim?
Type of Measure	Continuous
Reporting Value	90th Percentile
Continuous Variable Statement (Denominator Population)	Major Trauma Victims
Example of Final Reporting Value	11.6 mins
Numerator Statement (sub-population)	On scene time interval – wheel stop wheel go.
Indicator Formula Numeric Expression	1. Rank all values (time intervals) 2. Determine 90th percentile ranking value (x.90). Find 90% ranking and report that interval.
Suggested Display Format & Frequency	Column graph or process chart
Suggested Statistical Measures	☐ Mean ☐ Median ☐ Variance ☐ Mode ☐ Standard Deviation
Trending Analysis	■ Yes ☐ No
Benchmark Analysis	■ Yes ☐ No
References	1. 911 Dispatch data base

DISCLOSURE

Regarding these Indicator Specification Sheets

The following Indicator Specification Sheets were developed as part of a grant project executed in 2003. They are intended to be used as a **guide only**. These are original versions and in many cases have been updated and improved as they were implemented and used. They may also contain old information and possible some errors as they were not completely vetted or used by an official CQI representative body. They are best used as simply an example.

I include them for reference only in hopes that they may be helpful to have as a template or draft in order to enhance and stimulate the development of your own versions and based upon the consensus and standards of care in your community.

Indicator ID	*TR#C0001*	
Indicator Title	**% Major Trauma Victims**	
Objective	What percent (%) of all EMS transports are triaged to a trauma center?	
Type	Process	
Reporting Value and Units	Numeric Percentage (%)	
Define (Population) Denominator	Number of EMS transports	
Denominator Inclusion Criteria	**Criteria**	**Data Elements**
	1. Age 15 or older 2. Mode of transport via EMS ambulance 3. Incident occurred in	• Age • Mode of transport • EMS Call • Location County
Sub-population Numerator	Number of EMS transports triaged to Trauma Center	
Numerator Inclusion Criteria	**Criteria**	**Data Elements**
	1. Injury Severity Score of 15 or greater 2. Arrival at Trauma Center	• Trauma Alert • ISS • Arrival
Exclusion Criteria	*Criteria*	**Data Elements**
	1. Patients without mechanism of injury 2. Patients not transported to Trauma Center 3. Patients not Transported	• Mechanism of injury • Destination • Trauma triage decision
Indicator Formula Numeric Expression	The formula is to divide (/) the numerator (N) by the denominator (D) and then multiply (x) by 100 to obtain the (%) value the indicator is to report. Therefore the indicator expressed numerically is N/D =%	
Example of Final Reporting Value	10%	
Suggested Display Format Frequency	Process control or run chart by month	
Suggested Statistical Measure	Mean (x); Mode (m)	
Trending Analysis	Yes	
Benchmark Analysis	(TBD)	
Data Sources	Trauma One Registry/MEDS 3/ Business Objects/	

Indicator ID	TR#C0003	
Indicator Title	**% Discharged Home from ED - Quarterly**	
Objective	What percent (%) of major trauma victims which are triaged to a Trauma Center are discharged home from the Emergency Department alive?	
Type	Outcome	
Reporting Value and Units	Numeric Percentage (%)	
Define (Population) Denominator	Total EMS Activations.	
Denominator Inclusion Criteria	**Criteria**	**Data Elements**
	1. Age 15 or older 2. ISS of 15 or greater 3. Arrival by EMS ambulance 4. Arrival at Trauma Center	• Age • ISS • Mode of arrival • Arrival Time
Define (Sub Population) Numerator	Total EMS activations Discharged Home from ED (ED Disposition)	
Numerator Inclusion Criteria	**Criteria**	**Data Elements**
	1. Discharged alive form ED of TC	• Discharge Status
Exclusion Criteria	**Criteria**	**Data Elements**
	1. Patients not transported 2. Patients not transported to Trauma Center	• Destination
Indicator Formula Numeric Expression	The formula is to divide (/) the numerator (N) by the denominator (D) and then multiply (x) by 100 to obtain the (%) value the indicator is to report. Therefore the indicator expressed numerically is N/D =%	
Example of Final Reporting Value (number and units)	98%	
Suggested Display Format & Frequency	Process control or run chart by month	
Suggested Statistical Measures	Mean (x); Mode (m)	
Trending Analysis	Yes	
Benchmark Analysis	(TBD)	
Data Sources	MEDS 3/ Business Objects/Trauma One	
References	1. J Trauma. 1994 Oct;37(4):565-73; discussion 573-5. American College of Surgeons trauma quality indicators: an analysis of outcome in a statewide trauma registry. Nayduch D, Moylan J, Snyder BL, Andrews L, Rutledge R, Cunningham P. SourceDuke University Medical Center, Durham, NC 27710 2. Crit Care Med. 2011 Apr;39(4):846-59. Evidence for quality indicators to evaluate adult trauma care: a systematic review. Stelfox HT, Straus SE, Nathens A, Bobranska-Artiuch B. SourceDepartment of Critical Care Medicine, Medicine and Community Health Sciences, University of Calgary, Calgary, Alberta, Canada. tstelfox@ucalgary.ca Core Performance Measures: Stroke; NEMSIS.Core Indicators: CEMSIS. 3. NEMSIS Core Measures – Trauma 4. CEMSIS Core Measures – Trauma Center Criteria	

Indicator ID	TR#C0005
Indicator Title	**% Helicopter Transport - Quarterly**
Objective	What percent (%) of all MTV are transported by Air Ambulance?
Type	Process
Reporting Value and Units	Numeric Percentage (%)
Define (Population) Denominator	Total number of patients with ISS >15 transports from scene

Denominator Inclusion Criteria	Criteria	Data Elements
	1. Patients with ISS > 15 2. Time period by Quarter	• Date • ISS • Transports

Define (Sub-Population) Numerator	Total number of patients with ISS > 15 transported by air from scene

Numerator Inclusion Criteria	Criteria	Data Elements
	1. Transported by air ambulance	• Transport time • Air ambualnce

Exclusion Criteria	Criteria	Data Elements
	1. Non Transports 2. Non Air (ground) transports 3. ISS < 15	• Ground transports • ISS

Indicator Formula Numeric Expression	The formula is to divide total numerator (N) values by the total denominator (D) values and then multiply (x) by 100 to obtain the (%) value the indicator is to report. Therefore the indicator expressed numerically is N/D =% Median Time
Example of Final Reporting Value (number and units)	100%
Suggested Display Format & Frequency	Process Control by Month
Suggested Statistical Measures	NA
Trending Analysis	Yes by month as needed.
Benchmark Analysis	(TBD)
Data Sources	Reddinet
References	1. NEMSIS Core Measures – Trauma 2. CEMSIS Core Measures – Trauma Center Criteria

Revised – Version 2: 10/13/11

Indicator ID	TR#C0010
Indicator Title	**% Scene Time Interval (11-20 mins)- Hypotensive Major Trauma Victim**
Objective	In Contra Costa County, what percent (%) of adult hypotensive major trauma victims, have a Prehospital scene time interval of 10 minutes or less
Type	Process
Reporting Value and Units	% 0-10 mins
Define Denominator	All patients 15 years or older who are documented by EMS as major trauma victim (MTV) who arrive via EMS at a trauma Center.

Denominator Inclusion Criteria	Criteria	Data Elements
	1. Age 15 or older 2. Injury Severity Score of 15 or greater 3. Blood Pressure less than 90 mm 4. Mode of arrival via EMS 5. Incident occurred in	• Age • Trauma Alert • ISS • BP<90 • Mode of Arrival • Location County

Define Numerator	Times on scene from arrival is between eleven (11) and twenty (20) minutes

Numerator Inclusion Criteria	Criteria	Data Elements
	1. Lapsed Time (Arrival-Departure) on Scene in minutes	• Arrival time in minutes • Departure time in minutes

Exclusion Criteria	Criteria	Data Elements
	1. Patients not transported 2. Patients not transported to Trauma Center	

Indicator Formula Numeric Expression	The formula is to divide (/) the numerator (N) by the denominator (D) and then multiply (x) by 100 to obtain the (%) value the indicator is to report. Therefore the indicator expressed numerically is N/D =%
Example of Final Reporting Value (number and units)	98%
Suggested Display Format & Frequency	Process control or run chart by month
Suggested Statistical Measures	Mean (x); Mode (m)
Trending Analysis	Yes
Benchmark Analysis	(TBD)
Data Sources	MEDS 3/ Business Objects/Trauma One
References	1. J Trauma. 1994 Oct;37(4):565-73; discussion 573-5. American College of Surgeons trauma quality indicators: an analysis of outcome in a statewide trauma registry. Nayduch D, Moylan J, Snyder BL, Andrews L, Rutledge R, Cunningham P. SourceDuke University Medical Center, Durham, NC 27710 2. Crit Care Med. 2011 Apr;39(4):846-59. Evidence for quality indicators to evaluate adult trauma care: a systematic review. Stelfox HT, Straus SE, Nathens A, Bobranska-Artiuch B. SourceDepartment of Critical Care Medicine, Medicine and Community Health Sciences, University of Calgary, Calgary, Alberta, Canada. tstelfox@ucalgary.ca Core Performance Measures: Stroke; NEMSIS.Core Indicators: CEMSIS. 3. NEMSIS Core Measures – Trauma 4. CEMSIS Core Measures – Trauma Center Criteria

Revised – Version 2: 10/13/11

Indicator ID	**TR#C0001**
Indicator Title	**% Under-Triage Quarterly**
Objective	What percent (%) of adult major trauma victims are not triaged to a Trauma Center?
Type	Process
Reporting Value and Units	Numeric Percentage (%)
Define (Population) Denominator	Number of EMS activations with ISS >15 and number of triages to receiving facilities >15 = total under-triage. .

Denominator Inclusion Criteria	**Criteria**	**Data Elements**
	1. Age 15 or older 2. Mechanism of injury 3. Mode of arrival via EMS ambulance 4. Incident occurred in	• Age • Mechanism of Injury • Mode of Arrival • Location County

Define (Sub-population) Numerator	Number of under triages ISS .15 .

Numerator Inclusion Criteria	**Criteria**	**Data Elements**
	1. Injury Severity Score of 15 or greater	• Trauma Alert • ISS

Exclusion Criteria	**Criteria**	**Data Elements**
	1. Patients without mechanism of injury 2. Patients transported to Trauma Center 3. Patients not Transported	• Mechanism of injury • Destination •

Indicator Formula Numeric Expression	The formula is to divide (/) the numerator (N) by the denominator (D) and then multiply (x) by 100 to obtain the (%) value the indicator is to report. Therefore the indicator expressed numerically is N/D =%
Example of Final Reporting Value (number and units)	98%
Suggested Display Format & Frequency	Process control or run chart by month
Suggested Statistical Measures	Mean (x); Mode (m)
Trending Analysis	Yes
Benchmark Analysis	(TBD)
Data Sources	Trauma One Registry/MEDS 3/ Business Objects/
References	1. J Trauma. 1994 Oct;37(4):565-73; discussion 573-5. American College of Surgeons trauma quality indicators: an analysis of outcome in a statewide trauma registry. Nayduch D, Moylan J, Snyder BL, Andrews L, Rutledge R, Cunningham P. SourceDuke University Medical Center, Durham, NC 27710 2. Crit Care Med. 2011 Apr;39(4):846-59. Evidence for quality indicators to evaluate adult trauma care: a systematic review. Stelfox HT, Straus SE, Nathens A, Bobranska-Artiuch B. SourceDepartment of Critical Care Medicine, Medicine and Community Health Sciences, University of Calgary, Calgary, Alberta, Canada. tstelfox@ucalgary.ca Core Performance Measures: Stroke; NEMSIS.Core Indicators: CEMSIS. 3. NEMSIS Core Measures – Trauma 4. CEMSIS Core Measures – Trauma Center Criteria

Indicator ID	TR#C0002		
Indicator Title	**% Over-Triage Quarterly**		
Objective	In Contra Costa County, what percent (%) of non- major trauma victims are triaged to a Trauma Center		
Type	Process		
Reporting Value and Units	Numeric Percentage (%)		
Define (Population) Denominator	Number of EMS activations with ISS<15 and number of triages to receiving facilities ISS < 15 = total under-triage.		
Denominator Inclusion Criteria	**Criteria**		**Data Elements**
	1. Age 15 or older 2. Injury Severity Score of 15 or greater 3. Blood Pressure less than 90 mm 4. Mode of arrival via EMS 5. Incident occurred in		• Age • Trauma Alert • ISS • BP<90 • Mode of Arrival • Location County
Define (Sub-population) Numerator	Number of EMS activations with ISS<15		
Numerator Inclusion Criteria	**Criteria**		**Data Elements**
	1. Lapsed Time (Arrival-Departure) on Scene in minutes		• Arrival time in minutes • Departure time in minutes
Exclusion Criteria	**Criteria**		**Data Elements**
	1. Patients not transported 2. Patients not transported to TraumaCenter		
Indicator Formula Numeric Expression	The formula is to divide (/) the numerator (N) by the denominator (D) and then multiply (x) by 100 to obtain the (%) value the indicator is to report. Therefore the indicator expressed numerically is N/D =%		
Example of Final Reporting Value (number and units)	98%		
Suggested Display Format & Frequency	Process control or run chart by month		
Suggested Statistical Measures	Mean (x); Mode (m)		
Trending Analysis	Yes		
Benchmark Analysis	(TBD)		
Data Sources	MEDS 3/ Business Objects/Trauma One		
References	1. J Trauma. 1994 Oct;37(4):565-73; discussion 573-5. American College of Surgeons trauma quality indicators: an analysis of outcome in a statewide trauma registry. Nayduch D, Moylan J, Snyder BL, Andrews L, Rutledge R, Cunningham P. SourceDuke University Medical Center, Durham, NC 27710 2. Crit Care Med. 2011 Apr;39(4):846-59. Evidence for quality indicators to evaluate adult trauma care: a systematic review. Stelfox HT, Straus SE, Nathens A, Bobranska-Artiuch B. SourceDepartment of Critical Care Medicine, Medicine and Community Health Sciences, University of Calgary, Calgary, Alberta, Canada. tstelfox@ucalgary.ca Core Performance Measures: Stroke; NEMSIS.Core Indicators: CEMSIS. 3. NEMSIS Core Measures – Trauma 4. CEMSIS Core Measures – Trauma Center Criteria		

113

Indicator ID	STE#C0001
Indicator Title	**% EMS Scene Time (0-15) mins – STEMI**
Objective	What percent (%) of STEMI alert patients have a time interval between (0-15) mins from time of arrival to time of departure from scene by EMS transporting unit?
Type	Process
Reporting Value and Units	% 0-15 mins
Define Denominator	All patients 15 years or older who are documented by EMS as a STEMI Alert

Denominator Inclusion Criteria	Criteria	Data Elements
	1. Age 15 or older 2. STEMI Alert 3. Mode of arrival via EMS 4. Incident occurred in	• Age • STEMI Alert • Mode of Arrival • Location County

Define Numerator	Number of STEMI patients with scene time Intervals between zero (0) and fifteen (15) minutes

Numerator Inclusion Criteria	Criteria	Data Elements
	1. Lapsed times (on scene) in minutes 2. Difference of departure – arrival times in mins= 15 mins or less	• Time of arrival on scene in Mins • Time of departure from scene in mins

Exclusion Criteria	Criteria	Data Elements
	1. Patients not transported 2. Patients not triaged as STEMI Alert	

Indicator Formula Numeric Expression	The formula is to divide (/) the numerator (N) by the denominator (D) and then multiply (x) by 100 to obtain the (%) value the indicator is to report. Therefore the indicator expressed numerically is N/D =%
Example of Final Reporting Value (number and units)	98%
Suggested Display Format & Frequency	Process control or run chart by month
Suggested Statistical Measures	Mean (x); Mode (m)
Trending Analysis	Yes
Benchmark Analysis	(TBD)
Data Sources	MEDS 3/ Business Objects/STEMI
References	1. American Heart Association. Heart Disease and Stroke Statistics—2004 Update. Dallas, TX: American Heart Association 2003. 2. Best Practices in STEMI Management: The Cross Roads of Bleeding and Outcomes Condition: ACS; Ph. Gabriel Steg, MD; Anthony H. Gershlick, MBBS; Martial Hamon, MD, FESC; Authors and Disclosures; CME Released: 02/05/2010; Valid for credit through 02/05/2011 3. Mehta RH, Montoye CK, Gallogly M, et al., for the GAP Steering Committee of the American College of Cardiology. Improving quality of care for acute myocardial infarction: The Guidelines Applied in Practice (GAP) Initiative. JAMA. 2002; 287: 1269–1276. 4. NEMSIS Core Measures – STEMI 5. CEMSIS Core Measures – STEMI

Indicator ID	STE#C0002
Indicator Title	**% 911 Call to PCI (0-90) mins – STEMI**
Objective	What percent (%) of STEMI alert patients have a time interval between (0-90) mins from time 911 called and hospital intervention (PCI) ?
Type	Process
Reporting Value and Units	% 0-90 mins
Define Denominator	All patients 15 years or older who are documented by EMS as a STEMI Alert

Denominator Inclusion Criteria	Criteria	Data Elements
	1. Age 15 or older 2. STEMI Alert 3. Mode of arrival via EMS 4. Incident occurred in	• Age • STEMI Alert • Mode of Arrival • Location County

Define Numerator	Number of STEMI patients with scene time Intervals between zero (0) and fifteen (15) minutes

Numerator Inclusion Criteria	Criteria	Data Elements
	1. Lapsed Time (911-PCI)=90 mins or less 2. Time 911 call received – time hospital intervention=lapsed time interval	• Time of 911 received • Time hospital intervention PCI

Exclusion Criteria	Criteria	Data Elements
	1. Patients not transported 2. Patients not triaged as STEMI Alert	

Indicator Formula Numeric Expression	The formula is to divide (/) the numerator (N) by the denominator (D) and then multiply (x) by 100 to obtain the (%) value the indicator is to report. Therefore the indicator expressed numerically is N/D =%
Example of Final Reporting Value (number and units)	98%
Suggested Display Format & Frequency	Process control or run chart by month
Suggested Statistical Measures	Mean (x); Mode (m)
Trending Analysis	Yes
Benchmark Analysis	(TBD)
Data Sources	MEDS 3/ Business Objects/STEMI
References	1. American Heart Association. Heart Disease and Stroke Statistics—2004 Update. Dallas, TX: American Heart Association 2003. 2. Best Practices in STEMI Management: The Cross Roads of Bleeding and Outcomes Condition: ACS; Ph. Gabriel Steg, MD; Anthony H. Gershlick, MBBS; Martial Hamon, MD, FESC; Authors and Disclosures; CME Released: 02/05/2010; Valid for credit through 02/05/2011 3. Mehta RH, Montoye CK, Gallogly M, et al., for the GAP Steering Committee of the American College of Cardiology. Improving quality of care for acute myocardial infarction: The Guidelines Applied in Practice (GAP) Initiative. JAMA. 2002; 287: 1269–1276. 4. NEMSIS Core Measures – STEMI 5. CEMSIS Core Measures - STEMI

Indicator ID	STE#C0003
Indicator Title	**% Door to Intervention PCI in (0-60 mins) – STEMI**
Objective	What percent (%) of STEMI alert patients transported by EMS to a STEMI Center have a (in-hospital) door to intervention PCI time interval of (0-60) mins?
Type	Process
Reporting Value and Units	% 0-60 mins
Define Denominator	All patients 15 years or older who are documented by EMS as a STEMI Alert and transported to a STEMI facility

Denominator Inclusion Criteria	Criteria	Data Elements
	1. Age 15 or older 2. STEMI Alert 3. Mode of arrival to via EMS 4. Transported to STEMI Center 5. Incident occurred in	• Age • STEMI Alert • Mode of Arrival • STEMI Center • Location County

Define Numerator	Number of STEMI patients with scene time Intervals between zero (0) and fifteen (15) minutes

Numerator Inclusion Criteria	Criteria	Data Elements
	1. STEMI Patients 2. Lapsed Time = (arrival at hospital to PCI) in minutes	• STEMI • Time of arrival at hospital • Time of PCI intervention

Exclusion Criteria	Criteria	Data Elements
	1. Patients not transported 2. Patients not triaged as STEMI Alert 3. Lapse intervals > 60 mins	

Indicator Formula Numeric Expression	The formula is to divide (/) the numerator (N) by the denominator (D) and then multiply (x) by 100 to obtain the (%) value the indicator is to report. Therefore the indicator expressed numerically is N/D =%
Example of Final Reporting Value (number and units)	98%
Suggested Display Format & Frequency	Process control or run chart by month
Suggested Statistical Measures	Mean (x); Mode (m)
Trending Analysis	Yes
Benchmark Analysis	(TBD)
Data Sources	MEDS 3/ Business Objects/STEMI

Indicator ID	ST#C0001
Indicator Title	**% ARRIVAL AT STROKE CENTER < 60 MINS OF 911 CALL**
Objective	What percent (%) of adult patients who have a stroke reach the stroke center within sixty (60) minutes of calling 911?
Type	Process
Reporting Value and Units	% < 60 mins
Define Denominator	All patients 15 years or older who are documented by EMS as a stroke alert and who arrive via EMS at a Stroke Center.

Denominator Inclusion Criteria	Criteria	Data Elements
	1. Age 15 or older 2. Documented Stroke Alert patient 3. Mode of arrival via EMS 4. Incident occurred in	• Age • Stroke Alert • Mode of Arrival • Location County

Define Numerator	Times on scene from arrival to departure is less than sixty (60) minutes

Numerator Inclusion Criteria	Criteria	Data Elements
	1. Lapsed Time (Departure-Arrival) on Scene in minutes	• Departure Time in minutes • Arrival Time in minutes

Exclusion Criteria	Criteria	Data Elements
	1. Patients not transported 2. Patients not transported to Stroke Center	

Indicator Formula Numeric Expression	The formula is to divide (/) the numerator (N) by the denominator (D) and then multiply (x) by 100 to obtain the (%) value the indicator is to report. Therefore the indicator expressed numerically is N/D =%
Example of Final Reporting Value (number and units)	98%
Suggested Display Format & Frequency	Process control or run chart by month
Suggested Statistical Measures	Mean (x); Mode (m)
Trending Analysis	Yes
Benchmark Analysis	(TBD)
Data Sources	MEDS 3/ Business Objects
References	1. AHA/ASA Policy Statement; Implementation Strategies for Emergency Medical Services Within Stroke Systems of Care; A Policy Statement From the American Heart Association/ American Stroke Association Expert Panel on Emergency Medical Services Systems and the Stroke Council 2. Guidelines for the Primary Prevention of Stroke: A Guideline for Healthcare Professionals From the American Heart Association/American Stroke Association; Stroke. 2011;42:517-584, 3. Development of Stroke Performance Measures: Definitions, Methods, and Current Measures Stroke. AHA Stroke 2010;41:1573-1578, 4. Core Performance Measures: Stroke; NEMSIS. 5. Core Indicators: CEMSIS.

Indicator ID	ST#C002
Indicator Title	**% ARRIVAL AT STROKE CENTER 61 to 180 MINS OF 911 CALL**
Objective	What percent (%) of adult patients who have a stroke reach the stroke center within sixty (60) minutes of calling 911?
Type	Process
Reporting Value and Units	% between 61 to 180 mins
Define Denominator	All patients 15 years or older who are documented by EMS as a stroke alert and who arrive via EMS at a Stroke Center.

Denominator Inclusion Criteria	Criteria	Data Elements
	1. Age 15 or older 2. Documented Stroke Alert patient 3. Mode of arrival via EMS 4. Incident occurred in	• Age • Stroke Alert • Mode of Arrival • Location County

Define Numerator	Times on scene from arrival to departure is less than sixty (60) minutes

Numerator Inclusion Criteria	Criteria	Data Elements
	1. Lapsed Time (Departure-Arrival) on Scene in minutes	• Departure Time in minutes • Arrival Time in minutes

Exclusion Criteria	Criteria	Data Elements
	1. Patients not transported 2. Patients not transported to Stroke Center	

Indicator Formula Numeric Expression	The formula is to divide (/) the numerator (N) by the denominator (D) and then multiply (x) by 100 to obtain the (%) value the indicator is to report. Therefore the indicator expressed numerically is N/D =%
Example of Final Reporting Value (number or units)	90%
Suggested Display Format & Frequency	Process control or run chart by month
Suggested Statistical Measures	Mean (x); Mode (m)
Trending Analysis	Yes
Benchmark Analysis	(TBD)
Data Sources	MEDS 3/ Business Objects Data Systems
References	1. AHA/ASA Policy Statement; Implementation Strategies for Emergency Medical Services Within Stroke Systems of Care; A Policy Statement From the American Heart Association/ American Stroke Association Expert Panel on Emergency Medical Services Systems and the Stroke Council 2. Guidelines for the Primary Prevention of Stroke: A Guideline for Healthcare Professionals From the American Heart Association/American Stroke Association; Stroke. 2011;42:517-584, 3. Development of Stroke Performance Measures: Definitions, Methods, and Current Measures Stroke. AHA Stroke 2010;41:1573-1578, 4. Core Performance Measures: Stroke; NEMSIS. 5. Core Indicators: CEMSIS.

Indicator ID	ST#C0003
Indicator Title	**% Stroke Scene Time Interval (0-10 mins)**
Objective	What percent (%) of adult patients who have signs and symptoms of stroke, have a Prehospital scene time interval of 10 minutes or less
Type	Process
Reporting Value and Units	% 0-10 mins
Define Denominator	All patients 15 years or older who are documented by EMS as a stroke alert and who arrive via EMS at a Stroke Center.

Denominator Inclusion Criteria	Criteria	Data Elements
	1. Age 15 or older 2. Documented Stroke Alert patient 3. Mode of arrival via EMS 4. Incident occurred in	• Age • Stroke Alert • Mode of Arrival • Location County

Define Numerator	Times on scene from arrival is between zero (0) and ten (10) minutes

Numerator Inclusion Criteria	Criteria	Data Elements
	1. Lapsed Time (Arrival-Departure) on Scene in minutes	• Arrival time in minutes • Departure time in minutes

Exclusion Criteria	Criteria	Data Elements
	1. Patients not transported 2. Patients not transported to Stroke Center	

Indicator Formula Numeric Expression	The formula is to divide (/) the numerator (N) by the denominator (D) and then multiply (x) by 100 to obtain the (%) value the indicator is to report. Therefore the indicator expressed numerically is N/D =%
Example of Final Reporting Value (number and units)	98%
Suggested Display Format & Frequency	Process control or run chart by month
Suggested Statistical Measures	Mean (x); Mode (m)
Trending Analysis	Yes
Benchmark Analysis	(TBD)
Data Sources	MEDS 3/ Business Objects/Trauma One
References	1. AHA/ASA Policy Statement; Implementation Strategies for Emergency Medical Services Within Stroke Systems of Care; A Policy Statement From the American Heart Association/ American Stroke Association Expert Panel on Emergency Medical Services Systems and the Stroke Council 2. Guidelines for the Primary Prevention of Stroke: A Guideline for Healthcare Professionals From the American Heart Association/American Stroke Association; Stroke. 2011;42:517-584, 3. Development of Stroke Performance Measures: Definitions, Methods, and Current Measures Stroke. AHA Stroke 2010;41:1573-1578, 4. Core Performance Measures: Stroke; NEMSIS. 5. Core Indicators: CEMSIS.

Indicator ID	ST#C0004
Indicator Title	**% Stroke Scene Time Interval (11-15 mins)**
Objective	What percent (%) of adult patients who have signs and symptoms of stroke, have a Prehospital scene time interval of 10 minutes or less
Type	Process
Reporting Value and Units	% 11-15 mins
Define Denominator	All patients 15 years or older who are documented by EMS as a stroke alert and who arrive via EMS at a Stroke Center.

Denominator Inclusion Criteria	Criteria	Data Elements
	1. Age 15 or older 2. Documented Stroke Alert patient 3. Mode of arrival via EMS 4. Incident occurred in	• Age • Stroke Alert • Mode of Arrival • Location County

Define Numerator	Times on scene from arrival is between eleven (11) and fifteen (15) minutes

Numerator Inclusion Criteria	Criteria	Data Elements
	1. Lapsed Time (Arrival-Departure) on Scene in minutes	• Arrival time in minutes • Departure time in minutes

Exclusion Criteria	Criteria	Data Elements
	1. Patients not transported 2. Patients not transported to Stroke Center	

Indicator Formula Numeric Expression	The formula is to divide (/) the numerator (N) by the denominator (D) and then multiply (x) by 100 to obtain the (%) value the indicator is to report. Therefore the indicator expressed numerically is N/D =%
Example of Final Reporting Value (number and units)	98%
Suggested Display Format & Frequency	Process control or run chart by month
Suggested Statistical Measures	Mean (x); Mode (m)
Trending Analysis	Yes
Benchmark Analysis	(TBD)
Data Sources	MEDS 3/ Business Objects
References	1. AHA/ASA Policy Statement; Implementation Strategies for Emergency Medical Services Within Stroke Systems of Care; A Policy Statement From the American Heart Association/ American Stroke Association Expert Panel on Emergency Medical Services Systems and the Stroke Council 2. Guidelines for the Primary Prevention of Stroke: A Guideline for Healthcare Professionals From the American Heart Association/American Stroke Association; Stroke. 2011;42:517-584, 3. Development of Stroke Performance Measures: Definitions, Methods, and Current Measures Stroke. AHA Stroke 2010;41:1573-1578, 4. Core Performance Measures: Stroke; NEMSIS. 5. Core Indicators: CEMSIS.

Indicator ID	ST#C0005
Indicator Title	**% Stroke Scene Time Interval (16-20 mins)**
Objective	What percent (%) of adult patients who have signs and symptoms of stroke, have a Prehospital scene time interval of 10 minutes or less
Type	Process
Reporting Value and Units	% 16-20 mins
Define Denominator	All patients 15 years or older who are documented by EMS as a stroke alert and who arrive via EMS at a Stroke Center.

Denominator Inclusion Criteria	Criteria	Data Elements
	1. Age 15 or older 2. Documented Stroke Alert patient 3. Mode of arrival via EMS 4. Incident occurred in	• Age • Stroke Alert • Mode of Arrival • Location County

Define Numerator	Times on scene from arrival is between sixteen (16) and twenty (20) minutes

Numerator Inclusion Criteria	Criteria	Data Elements
	1. Lapsed Time (Arrival-Departure) on Scene in minutes	• Arrival time in minutes • Departure time in minutes

Exclusion Criteria	Criteria	Data Elements
	1. Patients not transported 2. Patients not transported to Stroke Center	

Indicator Formula Numeric Expression	The formula is to divide (/) the numerator (N) by the denominator (D) and then multiply (x) by 100 to obtain the (%) value the indicator is to report. Therefore the indicator expressed numerically is N/D =%
Example of Final Reporting Value (number and units)	98%
Suggested Display Format & Frequency	Process control or run chart by month
Suggested Statistical Measures	Mean (x); Mode (m)
Trending Analysis	Yes
Benchmark Analysis	(TBD)
Data Sources	MEDS 3/ Business Objects
References	1. AHA/ASA Policy Statement; Implementation Strategies for Emergency Medical Services Within Stroke Systems of Care; A Policy Statement From the American Heart Association/ American Stroke Association Expert Panel on Emergency Medical Services Systems and the Stroke Council 2. Guidelines for the Primary Prevention of Stroke: A Guideline for Healthcare Professionals From the American Heart Association/American Stroke Association; Stroke. 2011;42:517-584, 3. Development of Stroke Performance Measures: Definitions, Methods, and Current Measures Stroke. AHA Stroke 2010;41:1573-1578, 4. Core Performance Measures: Stroke; NEMSIS. 5. Core Indicators: CEMSIS.

Indicator ID	ST#C0006
Indicator Title	**% Stroke Center Door to Needle (0-60 mins)**
Objective	What percent (%) of adult patients who are assessed and transported to a stroke center as stroke alert have a door to needle time interval of 60 minutes or less
Type	Process
Reporting Value and Units	% 0-60 mins
Define Denominator	All patients 15 years or older who are documented by EMS as a stroke alert and who arrive via EMS at a Stroke Center.

Denominator Inclusion Criteria	Criteria	Data Elements
	1. Age 15 or older 2. Documented Stroke Alert patient 3. Mode of arrival via EMS 4. Incident occurred in	• Age • Stroke Alert • Mode of Arrival • Location County

Define Numerator	Number of patients whose door to needle time interval at Stroke Center was documented to be between zero (0) and ten (10) minutes

Numerator Inclusion Criteria	Criteria	Data Elements
	1. Lapsed Time in minutes (Arrival at Center –needle insertion with intent of administering ant-coagulant therapy)	• Arrival at stroke center time in minutes • Needle insertion time in minutes

Exclusion Criteria	Criteria	Data Elements
	1. Patients not transported 2. Patients not transported to Stroke Center	

Indicator Formula Numeric Expression	The formula is to divide (/) the numerator (N) by the denominator (D) and then multiply (x) by 100 to obtain the (%) value the indicator is to report. Therefore the indicator expressed numerically is N/D =%
Example of Final Reporting Value (number and units)	50%
Suggested Display Format & Frequency	Process control or run chart by month
Suggested Statistical Measures	Mean (x); Mode (m)
Trending Analysis	Yes
Benchmark Analysis	(TBD)
Data Sources	California Stroke Registry
References	1. AHA/ASA Policy Statement; Implementation Strategies for Emergency Medical Services Within Stroke Systems of Care; A Policy Statement From the American Heart Association/ American Stroke Association Expert Panel on Emergency Medical Services Systems and the Stroke Council 2. Guidelines for the Primary Prevention of Stroke: A Guideline for Healthcare Professionals From the American Heart Association/American Stroke Association; Stroke. 2011;42:517-584, 3. Development of Stroke Performance Measures: Definitions, Methods, and Current Measures Stroke. AHA Stroke 2010;41:1573-1578, 4. Core Performance Measures: Stroke; NEMSIS. 5. Core Indicators: CEMSIS.

Indicator ID	ST#C0007
Indicator Title	**% Stroke Center Door to Needle (61-120 mins)**
Objective	What percent (%) of adult patients who are assessed and transported to a stroke center as stroke alert have a door to needle time interval of 60 minutes or less
Type	Process
Reporting Value and Units	% 61-120 mins
Define Denominator	All patients 15 years or older who are documented by EMS as a stroke alert and who arrive via EMS at a Stroke Center.

Denominator Inclusion Criteria	Criteria	Data Elements
	1. Age 15 or older 2. Documented Stroke Alert patient 3. Mode of arrival via EMS 4. Incident occurred in	• Age • Stroke Alert • Mode of Arrival • Location County

Define Numerator	Number of patients whose door to needle time interval at Stroke Center was documented to be between sixty one (61) and one hundred and twenty (120) minutes

Numerator Inclusion Criteria	Criteria	Data Elements
	1. Lapsed Time in minutes (Arrival at Center –needle insertion with intent of administering ant-coagulant therapy)	• Arrival at stroke center time in minutes • Needle insertion time in minutes

Exclusion Criteria	Criteria	Data Elements
	1. Patients not transported 2. Patients not transported to Stroke Center	

Indicator Formula Numeric Expression	The formula is to divide (/) the numerator (N) by the denominator (D) and then multiply (x) by 100 to obtain the (%) value the indicator is to report. Therefore the indicator expressed numerically is N/D =%
Example of Final Reporting Value (number and units)	50%
Suggested Display Format & Frequency	Process control or run chart by month
Suggested Statistical Measures	Mean (x); Mode (m)
Trending Analysis	Yes
Benchmark Analysis	(TBD)
Data Sources	California Stroke Registry
References	1. AHA/ASA Policy Statement; Implementation Strategies for Emergency Medical Services Within Stroke Systems of Care; A Policy Statement From the American Heart Association/ American Stroke Association Expert Panel on Emergency Medical Services Systems and the Stroke Council 2. Guidelines for the Primary Prevention of Stroke: A Guideline for Healthcare Professionals From the American Heart Association/American Stroke Association; Stroke. 2011;42:517-584, 3. Development of Stroke Performance Measures: Definitions, Methods, and Current Measures Stroke. AHA Stroke 2010;41:1573-1578, 4. Core Performance Measures: Stroke; NEMSIS. 5. Core Indicators: CEMSIS.

Indicator ID	ST#C0008
Indicator Title	**% Stroke Center Door to Needle (< 180 mins)**
Objective	What percent (%) of adult patients who are assessed and transported to a stroke center as stroke alert have a door to needle time interval of 180 minutes or less
Type	Process
Reporting Value and Units	% <180 mins
Define Denominator	All patients 15 years or older who are documented by EMS as a stroke alert and who arrive via EMS at a Stroke Center.

Denominator Inclusion Criteria	**Criteria**	**Data Elements**
	1. Age 15 or older 2. Documented Stroke Alert patient 3. Mode of arrival via EMS 4. Incident occurred in County	• Age • Stroke Alert • Mode of Arrival • Location County

Define Numerator	Number of patients whose door to needle time interval at Stroke Center was documented to be one hundred and eighty (180) minutes or less.

Numerator Inclusion Criteria	**Criteria**	**Data Elements**
	1. Lapsed Time in minutes (Arrival at Center –needle insertion with intent of administering ant-coagulant therapy)	• Arrival at stroke center time in minutes • Needle insertion time in minutes

Exclusion Criteria	**Criteria**	**Data Elements**
	1. Patients not transported 2. Patients not transported to Stroke Center	

Indicator Formula Numeric Expression	The formula is to divide (/) the numerator (N) by the denominator (D) and then multiply (x) by 100 to obtain the (%) value the indicator is to report. Therefore the indicator expressed numerically is N/D =%
Example of Final Reporting Value (number and units)	50%
Suggested Display Format & Frequency	Process control or run chart by month
Suggested Statistical Measures	Mean (x); Mode (m)
Trending Analysis	Yes
Benchmark Analysis	(TBD)
Data Sources	California Stroke Registry
References	1. AHA/ASA Policy Statement; Implementation Strategies for Emergency Medical Services Within Stroke Systems of Care; A Policy Statement From the American Heart Association/ American Stroke Association Expert Panel on Emergency Medical Services Systems and the Stroke Council 2. Guidelines for the Primary Prevention of Stroke: A Guideline for Healthcare Professionals From the American Heart Association/American Stroke Association; Stroke. 2011;42:517-584, 3. Development of Stroke Performance Measures: Definitions, Methods, and Current Measures Stroke. AHA Stroke 2010;41:1573-1578, 4. Core Performance Measures: Stroke; NEMSIS. 5. Core Indicators: CEMSIS.

Indicator ID	ST#C0009
Indicator Title	**% Stroke Alert Patients by Mode of Arrival**
Objective	What are the modes of arrival by percentage (%) for adult patients who are assessed as stroke alert patients by stoke centers?.
Type	Process
Reporting Value and Units	% EMS, POV, WI, Other
Define Denominator	All patients 15 years or older who are documented by EMS as a stroke alert and who arrive and are assessed as a stroke alert patient by the stroke center.

Denominator Inclusion Criteria	Criteria	Data Elements
	1. Age 15 or older 2. Documented Stroke Alert patient 3. Incident occurred in Contra Costa County	• Age • Stroke Alert • Location County

Define Numerator	MULTIPLE NUMERATORS 1. Number of patients whose mode of arrival was by EMS 2. Number of patients whose mode of arrival was by, Private Operated Vehicle (POV). 3. Number of patients whose mode of arrival was by Walk in (WI) 4. Number of patients whose mode of arrival was by Other means

Numerator Inclusion Criteria	Criteria	Data Elements
	1. Mode of Trans- EMS 2. Mode of Trans – POV 3. Mode of Trans – WI 4. Mode of Trans - Other	• Mode EMS • Mode POV • Mode WI • Mode Other

Exclusion Criteria	Criteria	Data Elements
	1. Patients not assessed as stroke alert in Stroke Center	

Indicator Formula Numeric Expression	The formula is to divide (/) the numerators individually (N) by the denominator (D) and then multiply (x) by 100 to obtain the (%) value the indicator is to report. Therefore the indicator expressed numerically is N/D =%
Example of Final Reporting Value (number and units)	% EMS % POV % WI % Other
Suggested Display Format & Frequency	Pie Chart - Quarterly
Suggested Statistical Measures	NA
Trending Analysis	Yes – could be stratified to run chart review
Benchmark Analysis	(TBD)
Data Sources	California Stroke Registry
References	1. AHA/ASA Policy Statement; Implementation Strategies for Emergency Medical Services Within Stroke Systems of Care; A Policy Statement From the American Heart Association/ American Stroke Association Expert Panel on Emergency Medical Services Systems and the Stroke Council 2. Guidelines for the Primary Prevention of Stroke: A Guideline for Healthcare Professionals From the American Heart Association/American Stroke Association; Stroke. 2011;42:517-584, 3. Development of Stroke Performance Measures: Definitions, Methods, and Current Measures Stroke. AHA Stroke 2010;41:1573-1578, 4. Core Performance Measures: Stroke; NEMSIS. 5. Core Indicators: CEMSIS.

Index ID	SU-C#0002
Indicator Title	**Number of 911 Transports**
Objective	What is the number of 911 patients transported to receiving facilities during a specific time interval?
Type	outcome
Reporting Value and Units	numeric per specified time period (time, dates, month, quarter year, semi-annual, annual)
Define Denominator (POPULATION)	Number of arrivals of 911 patients at receiving facilities

Denominator Inclusion Criteria	Criteria	Data Elements
	1. 911 call received by dispatch center 2. Arrivals at receiving facility with patient 3. Begin date 4. End date	• Call Received • Unit transporting • Unit Arrival • Month • Day • Year

Define Numerator (SUB POPULATION)	NA

Numerator Inclusion Criteria	Criteria	Data Elements
	1. NA	• NA

Exclusion Criteria	Criteria	Data Elements
	1. NA	• NA

Indicator Formula Numeric Expression	No formula required.
Example of Final Reporting Value (number and units)	5490 per specified time: i.e.; QTR 1 (Jan-Mar 2012)
Suggested Display Format & Frequency	run chart or bar chart by time period specified
Suggested Statistical Measures	Mean (x); Mode (m)
Trending Analysis	Optional
Benchmark Analysis	(TBD)
Data Sources	MEDS 3.0 and Zoll
References	1. NEMSIS Core Measures 2. CEMSIS Core Measures
Approval	Final: March 2012 IRC & QLC

Index ID	SU-C#0003
Indicator Title	**Customer Satisfaction – Overall**
Objective	What is the overall satisfaction level of patients who receive service from ambulance providers in County?
Type	outcome
Reporting Value and Units	numeric as expressed on a scale of agreement 1-5
Define Denominator (POPULATION)	Total patients who respond to survey by choosing values of 1-5 to express their level of satisfaction with the customer care given by ambulance provider.

Denominator Inclusion Criteria	Criteria	Data Elements
	1. Patients responding to customer surveys about level of satisfaction 2. Response of customer 1-5 weighted upon level of agreement	• Response 1-5 based upon level of agreement

Define Numerator (SUB POPULATION)		
Response 1. Strongly disagree		Response 2. Disagrees
Response 3. Neutral		Response 4. Agree
Response 5. Strongly Agree		

Numerator Inclusion Criteria	Criteria	Data Elements
	1. Responses to specific levels of agreement as defined above in numerator	• Strongly disagree • Disagree • Neutral • Agree • Strongly Disagree

Exclusion Criteria	Criteria	Data Elements
	1. NA	• NA

Indicator Formula Numeric Expression	No formula required.
Example of Final Reporting Value (number and units)	56 strongly agree; 32 agree; 12 neutral; 3 disagree; 1 strongly disagree
Suggested Display Format & Frequency	bar chart by time period specified
Suggested Statistical Measures	NA
Trending Analysis	Optional
Benchmark Analysis	(TBD)
Data Sources	Provider reports
References	1. NEMSIS Core Measures 2. CEMSIS Core Measures
Approval	Final: March 2012 CCCEMS IRC & QLC

Index ID	SU-C#0004
Indicator Title	**Number of Multi Casualty Incident Plan Activations**
Objective	What is the number of times the multi casualty incident plan was activated in County over a specific time interval?
Type	outcome
Reporting Value and Units	numeric per specified time period (time, dates, month, quarter, semi-annual, annual)
Define Denominator (POPULATION)	number of times the multi casualty incident plan was activated in County over a specific time interval.

Denominator Inclusion Criteria	Criteria	Data Elements
	1. MCI plan activated	• MCI

Define Numerator (SUB POPULATION)	NA	

Numerator Inclusion Criteria	Criteria	Data Elements
	1. NA	• NA

Exclusion Criteria	Criteria	Data Elements
	1. NA	• NA

Indicator Formula Numeric Expression	No formula required.
Example of Final Reporting Value (number and units)	5 per specified time: i.e.; QTR 1 (Jan-Mar 2012)
Suggested Display Format & Frequency	bar chart by time period specified
Suggested Statistical Measures	NA
Trending Analysis	Optional
Benchmark Analysis	(TBD)
Data Sources	ReddiNet
References	1. ReddiNet 2. OES 3. NEMSIS Core Measures 4. CEMSIS Core Measures
Approval	Final: March 2012 CCCEMS IRC & QLC

Index ID	SU-C#0001
Indicator Title	**Number of 911 Responses**
Objective	What is the number of 911 unit responses during a specific time interval?
Type	outcome
Reporting Value and Units	numeric per specified time period (time, dates, month, quarter year, semi-annual, annual)
Define Denominator (POPULATION)	Number of 911 calls received by a dispatch center where an EMS response unit (Transporting and/or non-transporting) is documented as responding to an emergency call for assistance, care or transportation.

Denominator Inclusion Criteria	Criteria	Data Elements
	1. 911 call received by dispatch center 2. EMS response unit documented as responding 3. Begin date 4. End date	• Call Received • Unit Dispatched • Unit Responding • Month • Day • Year

Define Numerator (SUB POPULATION)	NA

Numerator Inclusion Criteria	Criteria	Data Elements
	1. NA	• NA

Exclusion Criteria	Criteria	Data Elements
	1. NA	• NA

Indicator Formula Numeric Expression	No formula required.
Example of Final Reporting Value (number and units)	8,250 per specified time: ie; QTR 1 (Jan-Mar 2012)
Suggested Display Format & Frequency	run chart or bar chart by time period specified
Suggested Statistical Measures	Mean (x); Mode (m)
Trending Analysis	Optional
Benchmark Analysis	(TBD)
Data Sources	MEDS 3.0 and Zoll
References	1. NEMSIS Core Measures 2. CEMSIS Core Measures
Approval	Final: March 2012 IRC & QLC

Index ID	BH-C#0001		
Indicator Title	**Base Hospital Call Volume**		
Objective	What is the number of EMS calls received via radio or telecommunications by base hospitals over a specified time interval?		
Type	outcome		
Reporting Value and Units	numeric per specified time period (time, dates, month, quarter year, semi-annual, annual)		
Define Denominator (POPULATION)	the number of EMS calls received via radio or telecommunications by base hospitals over specified time interval		
Denominator Inclusion Criteria	**Criteria**		**Data Elements**
	1. EMS call received 2. Begin date 3. End date		• EMS call received • Month • Day • Year
Define Numerator (SUB POPULATION)	NA		
Numerator Inclusion Criteria	**Criteria**		**Data Elements**
	1. NA		• NA
Exclusion Criteria	**Criteria**		**Data Elements**
	1. NA		• NA
Indicator Formula Numeric Expression	No formula required.		
Example of Final Reporting Value (number and units)	450 calls per specified time: i.e.; QTR 1 (Jan-Mar 2012)		
Suggested Display Format & Frequency	run chart or bar chart by time period specified		
Suggested Statistical Measures	NA		
Trending Analysis	Optional		
Benchmark Analysis	(TBD)		
Data Sources	Base Hospital Log		
References	1. NEMSIS Core Measures 2. CEMSIS Core Measures		
Approval	Final: March 2012 CCCEMS IRC & QLC		

Index ID	BH-C#0002
Indicator Title	**Base Hospital Call Volume by Type**
Objective	What is the % trauma vs. medical types of EMS calls received via radio or telecommunications by base hospitals over a specified time interval?
Type	outcome
Reporting Value and Units	% Trauma % Medical
Define Denominator (POPULATION)	the number of EMS calls received via radio or telecommunications by base hospitals over specified time interval

Denominator Inclusion Criteria	Criteria	Data Elements
	1. EMS call received 2. Begin date 3. End date	• EMS call received • Month • Day • Year

Define Numerator (SUB POPULATION)	1. EMS calls identified as patients having traumatic mechanism of injury 2. EMS calls not identified as patients having a traumatic mechanism of injury

Numerator Inclusion Criteria	Criteria	Data Elements
	1. Patients with mechanism of injury	• Mechanism of injury

Exclusion Criteria	Criteria	Data Elements
	1. NA	• NA

Indicator Formula Numeric Expression	Divide (/) the numerator (N) by the denominator (D) and then multiply (x) by 100 to obtain the (%) value the indicator is to report. Therefore the indicator expressed numerically is N/D =%. . Medical is expressed as the remaining % subtracting trauma from 100%
Example of Final Reporting Value (number and units)	23% Trauma 77% Medical
Suggested Display Format & Frequency	Pie Chart
Suggested Statistical Measures	NA
Trending Analysis	Optional
Benchmark Analysis	NA
Data Sources	Base Hospital Log
References	1. NEMSIS Core Measures 2. CEMSIS Core Measures
Approval	Final: March 2012 CCCEMS IRC & QLC

Index ID	BH-C#0003		
Indicator Title	**Base Hospital Call Volume by Age**		
Objective	What is the % adult vs. pediatric ages for EMS calls received via radio or telecommunications by base hospitals over a specified time interval?		
Type	outcome		
Reporting Value and Units	% Adult % Pediatric		
Define Denominator (POPULATION)	the number of EMS calls received via radio or telecommunications by base hospitals over specified time interval		
Denominator Inclusion Criteria	**Criteria**		**Data Elements**
	1. EMS call received 2. Begin date 3. End date		• EMS call received • Month • Day • Year
Define Numerator (SUB POPULATION)	1. EMS calls identified as pediatric patients 2. EMS calls identified as adult patients		
Numerator Inclusion Criteria	**Criteria**		**Data Elements**
	1. EMS calls received by base hospital where patient has not yet reached the age of 14 years		• Age
Exclusion Criteria	**Criteria**		**Data Elements**
	1. Non EMS calls		• NA
Indicator Formula Numeric Expression	Divide (/) the numerator (N) by the denominator (D) and then multiply (x) by 100 to obtain the (%) value the indicator is to report. Therefore the indicator expressed numerically is N/D =%. . Adult is expressed as the remaining % subtracting pediatric from 100%		
Example of Final Reporting Value (number and units)	10% Pediatric 90% Adult		
Suggested Display Format & Frequency	Pie Chart		
Suggested Statistical Measures	NA		
Trending Analysis	Optional		
Benchmark Analysis	NA		
Data Sources	Base Hospital Log		
References	1. NEMSIS Core Measures 2. CEMSIS Core Measures		
Approval	Final: March 2012 CCCEMS IRC & QLC		

Index ID	PS-C#0001
Indicator Title	**Number of EMS Safety Events**
Objective	What is the number of EMS Patient Safety Events which occurred over a specified time interval?
Type	Outcome
Reporting Value and Units	numeric per specified time period interval
Define Denominator (POPULATION)	number of EMS Patient Safety Events which occurred over a specified time interval

Denominator Inclusion Criteria	Criteria	Data Elements
	1. Patient Safety Event Reported 2. Begin date 3. End date	• Event Entry • Month • Day • Year

Define Numerator (SUB POPULATION)	NA

Numerator Inclusion Criteria	Criteria	Data Elements
	1. NA	• NA

Exclusion Criteria	Criteria	Data Elements
	1. NA	• NA

Indicator Formula Numeric Expression	No formula required.
Example of Final Reporting Value (number and units)	18 events reported per QTR 1 (Jan-Mar 2012)
Suggested Display Format & Frequency	run chart or bar chart by time period specified
Suggested Statistical Measures	NA
Trending Analysis	Yes
Benchmark Analysis	(TBD)
Data Sources	Contra Costa County EMS EMS Events Reporting System
References	1. Policy #32; EMS Events Reporting Contra Costa EMS Policies & Procedures 2. NEMSIS Core Measures 3. CEMSIS Core Measures
Approval	Final: March 2012 CCCEMS IRC & QLC

Index ID	**PS-C#0002**	
Indicator Title	**EMS Safety Events by Clinical Issues**	
Objective	What is the top four (4) reported Clinical EMS Safety Events over a specified time interval?	
Type	outcome	
Reporting Value and Units	numeric	
Define Denominator (POPULATION)	Top four (4) most frequently occurring clinical categories as reported in the Contra Costa County EMS patient EMS Safety Events reporting system	
Denominator Inclusion Criteria	**Criteria**	**Data Elements**
	1. Event reported 2. Type of event	• Report entry • Type reported • Frequency of type • Rank of frequency
Define Numerator (SUB POPULATION)	1. Top four (4) events reported ranked by frequency	
Numerator Inclusion Criteria	**Criteria**	**Data Elements**
	1. Top four (4) based on frequency of reporting	• Type • Frquency
Exclusion Criteria	**Criteria**	**Data Elements**
	1. Not top 4 frequency	• Type • frequency
Indicator Formula Numeric Expression	No formula. Number only	
Example of Final Reporting Value (number and units)	Frequency ranked highest to lowest; I,e: assessment=10; airway=4; med=2; CPR=1	
Suggested Display Format & Frequency	Bar Chart	
Suggested Statistical Measures	Yes	
Trending Analysis	Yes	
Benchmark Analysis	NA	
Data Sources	Contra Costa County EMS EMS Events Reporting System	
References	1. Policy #32; EMS Events Reporting Contra Costa EMS Policies & Procedures 2. NEMSIS Core Measures 3. CEMSIS Core Measures	
Approval	Final: March 2012 CCCEMS IRC & QLC	

Index ID	PS-C#0003
Indicator Title	**EMS Safety Events by Operational Issues**
Objective	What is the top four (4) reported operational EMS Safety Events over a specified time interval?
Type	outcome
Reporting Value and Units	numeric
Define Denominator (POPULATION)	Top four (4) most frequently occurring operationall categories as reported in the Contra Costa County EMS patient EMS Safety Events reporting system

Denominator Inclusion Criteria	Criteria	Data Elements
	1. Event reported 2. Type of event 3. Operational	• Report entry • Type reported • Frequency of type • Rank of frequency

Define Numerator (SUB POPULATION)	1. Top four (4) events reported ranked by frequency	

Numerator Inclusion Criteria	Criteria	Data Elements
	1. Top four (4) operational based on frequency of reporting	• Type • Frequency

Exclusion Criteria	Criteria	Data Elements
	1. Not top 4 frequency operational	• Type • frequency

Indicator Formula Numeric Expression	No formula. Number only
Example of Final Reporting Value (number and units)	Frequency ranked highest to lowest; I,e: conductt=10; communications=4; destination=2; citizen complaint=1
Suggested Display Format & Frequency	Bar Chart
Suggested Statistical Measures	Yes
Trending Analysis	Yes
Benchmark Analysis	NA
Data Sources	Contra Costa County EMS EMS Events Reporting System
References	1. Policy #32; EMS Events Reporting Contra Costa EMS Policies & Procedures 2. NEMSIS Core Measures 3. CEMSIS Core Measures
Approval	Final: March 2012 CCCEMS IRC & QLC

About the Author

Craig Stroup is the director of the Center for Emergency Medical Services Performance Improvement and the author of many EMS articles and textbooks. He has extensive background and training in EMS systems, administration, quality improvement – especially the development and utilization of quality indicators as a powerful consensus and action tool.

With over 30 years of experience in EMS at all levels. He has been appointed and participated in many state and national EMS committees charged with developing programs and indicators for quality Improvement.
For more information or resources; Craig can be contacted at:
stroupems@msn.com

CEMSPI

Center for EMS Performance Improvement
www.cemspi.org

The Center for Emergency Medical Services (EMS) Performance improvement is a non-profit organization with the primary focus of advocating patient safety and system performance improvement specifically in the pre hospital setting.

CEMSPI works with many emergency medical services organizations to facilitate the collection, development, analysis, and maintenance of patient safety data and events reporting.

CEMSPI is also a leader in providing comprehensive quality improvement and patient safety consulting and many training options for EMS agencies and prehospital patient care providers.